Mentorship in Medicine

Bertha Chioma Ekeh

Cover image (Culled from htttps://www.dreamstime.com)

Copyright © 2018 Bertha Chioma Ekeh

All rights reserved.

ISBN: 978-1723719318
ISBN-13:978 1723719318

DEDICATION

TO THE ALMIGHTY GOD FROM WHOM ALL KNOWLEDGE COMES FROM

To all my Teachers and Mentors

And to you all reading this book who will benefit as either Mentors, Trainers or Mentees

CONTENT

1	Introduction	1
2	Types of Mentoring	10
3	Benefits of Mentorship	20
4	Medical Training in Nigeria	27
5	Mentorship in Medicine	31
6	Types of Mentors	41
7	The Mentoring Process	54
8	Challenges of Mentoring	65
9	The Myths of Mentorship	74
10	Starting off a Mentoring programme	83

FORWARD

"Mentorship in Medicine"
This title is a unique one- Hearing it announced for a CME (Continuing Medical Education) was not something that I wanted to miss. Hearing the presenter come out with a bang from the introduction made me glad that I was present. Listening through to the end, I thanked God for: both the Presenter and the Presentation.
"Put this in a book" and here it is! What an honour and priviledge she gave me to proof- read this wonderful book. I have learnt a couple of new words! The subject of Mentoring is so clearly brought to focus and well packaged in simple words for anyone to understand. We all resonate with this subject right from the home (via our parents especially our mothers) through school (via our teachers), to places of work where we meet with our bosses and co-workers. By the time you go through this book, you will certainly wish that it had come earlier for you to have been mentored better/harder.
The book is here now. It is not only for Doctors(Mentors and Mentees in the Mentoring Programmes of Residency Training), but it is for all who do not wish to die and be buried with those special gifts that God has blessed you with in whatever field. But rise higher by 'passing the baton" to the next generation.
Savour this book "Mentorship in Medicine" and get more copies as gifts to others.

Dr Mfon Edyang-Ekpa
BM, BCh. (UNN 1976), MPH (1981)
Pioneer HOD, Community Health Department: Sanni Abacha Specialist Hospital (Now UUTH Uyo)
Pioneer Focal Person for Anti Retroviral Drug Management South South zone Federal Medical Centre (Now UUTH Uyo), Nigeria

Reviews

Thank you for giving me the priviledge of this innovative read. I would strongly recommend it not only for all residents who wish to turn out successful, but also to all trainers. I find it a very interesting read.

Dr Christie Akwaowo
MBBCh, MSc. FMCPH, mHD–gN
President, Medical Women Association of Nigeria (MWAN),
Akwa Ibom State Branch 2017-2018 Biennium

If you want one year of prosperity, grow grain

If you want ten years of prosperity, grow trees

If you want one hundred years of prosperity, grow people.

- Chinese proverb

Mentorship is the key to extraordinary success

Mike Murdock

Mentorship in Medicine

ACKNOWLEDGEMENTS

I earnestly knowledge the following:

Dr Mfon Edyang- Ekpa
A renowned medical elder that encouraged me to write this book on Mentorship in Medicine.
Thank you Ma, this is solely your idea
You are my Cheerleader!

Dr Isaac Assam Udo sent me on this journey to study Mentorship. This book is as a result of that "assignment"
Thank you Sir!

Dr Christie Akwaowo spent valuable time from her hectic schedule to review this book.
Thank you my Presido!

CHAPTER 1

INTRODUCTION

"To see afar, you stand on the shoulders of giants"

Isaac Newton

This popular statement made by Isaac Newton many decades ago holds true till today. In any endeavour in life, it is often wiser to take the route of learning. The word mentor has always been used to denote a "father figure" who sponsors, guides and develops a younger person. Throughout history, mentors have played a significant role in teaching, inducting and developing the skills and talents of the young. Mentors are usually individuals who are known to be achievers. Most of us have undergone some form of mentoring which has guided and empowered us in our personal lives, marriages, raising our children and in our different professions. Recently however, Mentoring has been shown to be extremely important in businesses and professional development. It has been called the sine qua non of Management. In view of this, Mentoring is essential in every organization and profession including the Medical Profession. The essence of this book is to discuss the art and practice of mentoring (Mentorship) as it applies to the Medical Profession all over the world. It emanates for my passion to see exponential growth in the noble Medical Profession. In studying Mentoring, I have come to understand that Mentoring should also be the *sine qua non* for the Medical Profession.

Formal Mentoring is a new emerging concept in most

organizations and institutions. Most of what is written in this book is based on the little that I have learnt about mentoring (I am still learning) in medical practice albeit informally. It is my earnest desire and prayer that this book will be beneficial to every Doctor who is interested in mentoring and in being mentored: especially in Medical Training Programmes who hitherto had no Formal Mentoring Systems. This book will also benefit anyone who is interested in career development.

History of Mentorship

The word 'mentor' originates from Homer's classic poem; The Odyssey written in 800 BC. In this poem, Odyssey the king of Ithaca while preparing to leave for Troy appointed a guardian to look after his son Telemachus. The name of the guardian who acted in his place as teacher, advisor and friend was Mentor. It is from this story that the use of the word *mentor* as a wise and faithful counselor arose. *A mentor therefore is someone who is a counselor and a teacher who instructs, admonishes and assists a junior trainee or colleague in attaining success.*

Definition

There are several definitions of Mentoring. Two of them stand out in my opinion as follows:

Mentoring is a process for the informal transmission of knowledge, social capital, and the psychosocial support *perceived* by the recipient as relevant to work, career, or professional development; Mentoring entails informal communication, usually face-to-face and during a sustained period of time, between a person who is perceived to have greater relevant knowledge, wisdom, or experience (the mentor) and a person who is perceived to have less (the protégé, mentee, mentoree)". This book will use mentor and mentee in most instances. The cardinal issues in this definition are as follows:

1. Mentoring is a *process*; it is usually not a one–off experience. It lasts over a period of time and in some cases it lasts forever.
2. Mentoring involves an *informal* method of transmission. It usually does not require delivering of lectures, seminars or preaching: the environment is less formal and friendly.
3. The support is *perceived by the mentee as relevant* to work, career or professional development; any other information transmitted that is not applicable to career or professional development is not considered as part of the Mentoring.
4. The Mentoring process involves a *face-to-face communication*; the mentor is available to the mentee.
5. The *mentor must have greater knowledge experience or skill* than the mentee. These will be beneficial to the mentee.

The second definition I can relate with is -: "Mentoring is a learning relationship which helps people to take charge of their own development, to release their potential and to achieve results which they value."
This second definition still recognizes mentoring as a learning relationship but more importantly places *much emphasis on the resultant effect on the mentee*.
The salient features are as follows: The mentee *takes charge of his personal development*. This means that he is guided to take charge and not to remain the "Yes Man".
The Mentoring relationship helps the mentee to *release his personal innate potentials, qualities, passions and strengths*. The mentee is able to *achieve results which he or she values*. In essence, the mentee is the *eventual assessor of the mentoring relationship*.

Illustrations of Mentorship

1. Helping Hand

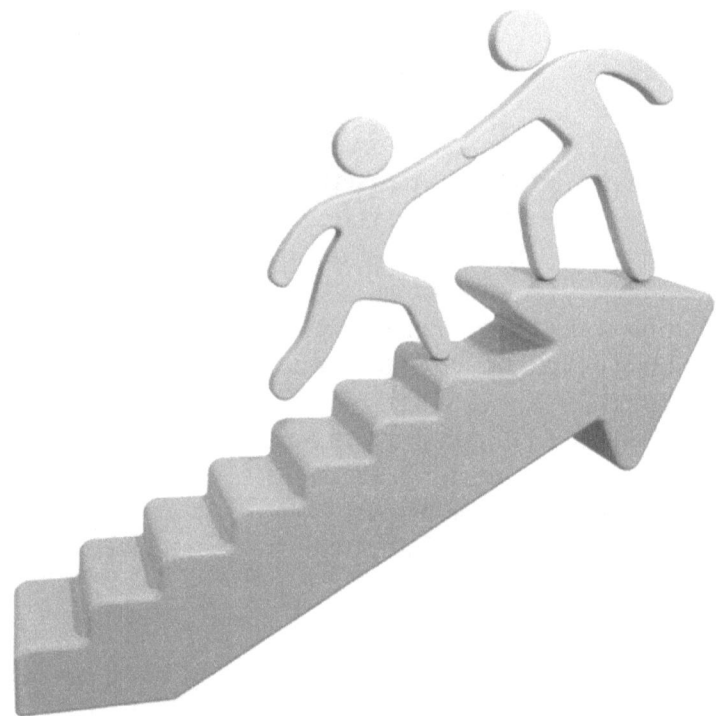

Fig1. Helping hand

(Culled from https://www.dreamstime.com)

One of my favourite illustrations of Mentoring is giving a helping hand as shown in Fig 1, above. The following facts are noted form this illustration:

1. The mentee is on the stair case *on his own volition and strength: not being carried by the Mentor*. The mentee does not expect everything to be done for him but has his own

intellect, ideas, innovations, will power and strength. In the Medical Profession, everyone goes through the ranks to get to the top. All the rungs on the ladder must be climbed; no one may take a leap or miss a step or two in order to get to the top of the ladder. The mentee therefore must exert energy to climb the ladder himself while the Mentor lends him a helping hand. Hence, the mentee is diligent, conscientious, ready and willing to pay the price.

2. The mentee is *on the right track* and moving in the right direction. He is focused on the job of climbing his career ladder successfully. Oh! He may take one or two wrong steps or stagger along the way. Nevertheless considering his determination, most likely he sure will get to the top of his career on his own but it will take a little more time. The mentor helps him to avoid some of the wrong steps and staggering.

In essence Mentoring is helping someone who is already standing, climbing the stair case, exerting energy, focused and moving in the right direction. Such a person will most likely get to the top with or without help. *When the Mentor lends him a helping hand, he has an easier, smoother and faster ride to finally stand on the same pedestal or podium with the mentor.*

The mentoring relationship is an essential step for achieving success in politics, business and academics. Indeed, most successful people in different areas of human endeavour can point to a mentor who was crucial to their career growth and success. The importance of mentoring throughout one's career has therefore been emphasized, especially during professional transitions.

2. Reproduction

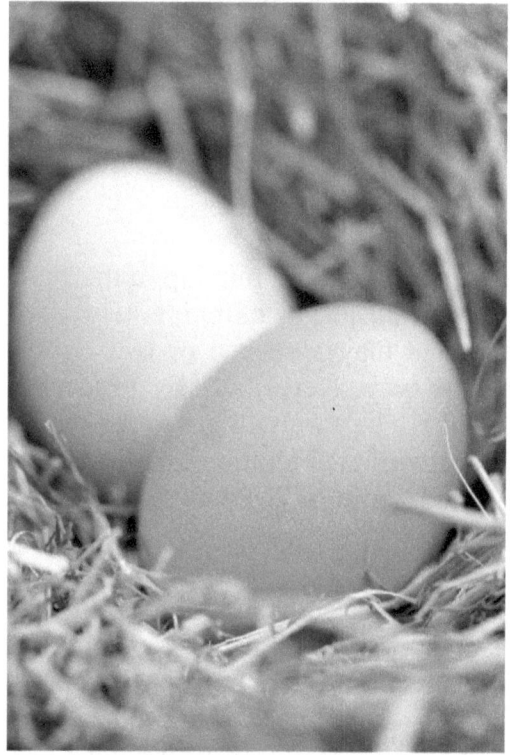

Fig 2. Reproduce like kind
(Culled from https://www.dreamstime.com)

One important characteristic of the living things as we all know is reproduction. Reproduction involves making another replica. Mentoring ensures that some of the qualities like the knowledge, skills, character, conduct and the passion for research are all replicated in the mentee. In essence, a Cardiologist should reproduce another Cardiologist; a Plastic Surgeon should reproduce another Plastic Surgeon and so on.

This is clearly written in the Holy Bible:
Ye shall know them by their fruits…… (Matt 7: 16-18).

Simple as this statement is, the basic truth remains that the fruit identifies the tree. There are many fruits that we know and eat but have never seen what the tree looks like. We can only identify such a tree when we see the fruit that it has borne hanging on it. The knowledge, skills and qualities in the mentees usually identify the mentor/trainer. The Histopathologist should not retire without producing another Histopathologist that is equally good or better than him; the Neurologist should not retire without having produced another Neurologist that is equally as good or even better and so on. *Mentoring aids the hospital, institution and Medical Profession as a whole to reproduce knowledge, skills, quality care and good character.*

The picture in fig 2 illustrates the characteristics of the reproduction that occurs within the mentoring relationship. The two eggs are exactly the same in terms of content, nutrients and all other features. *The two eggs have the same substance and serve exactly the same purpose.* They are used in the same dishes, baking, hatching chicks and others. However, there is a minor variation in colour. The mentor or trainer reproduces the most important aspects of himself or herself: the knowledge, skills, character, conduct, functions and or purpose are exactly the same. *However, their qualities, strengths, styles and approaches will differ to some extent. In essence, the mentor and mentee will be of different colours.*

3. Handing Over

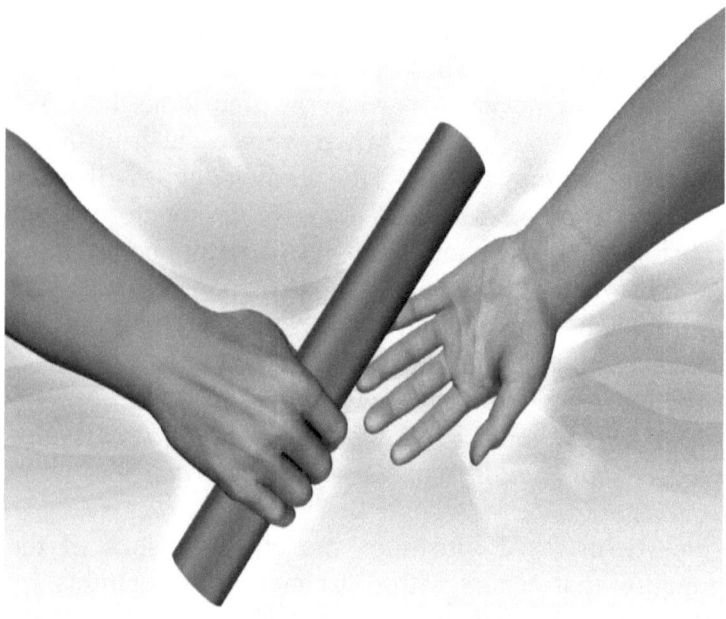

Fig3. Handing over
(Culled from https://www.dreamstime.com)

Another wonderful illustration of mentoring is *the handing over of the baton.* In a relay race, there are several sprinters. The success of the whole relay team is the success of all. Every sprinter in the team must run his lap well in order to achieve the eventual team success. *Most sprinters and Coaches consider the handing over of the baton the most critical aspect of the race.* Great teams have lost the race because the handing over was not properly done. Once the baton is dropped, the race is ruined and such teams never recover from the mishap. Therefore, the proper technique of handing over the baton is essential for the success of the relay race.

Mentoring can be illustrated as the mentor handing over the baton to the mentee to continue the race in which the mentor has run successfully till his own lap is completed. Once there is successful handing over of the baton, the success of the team is ensured. In mentoring therefore, the mentor gives a helping hand to the mentee who conscientiously climbs the career ladder till he can stand on the same pedestal with the mentor. In essence, the mentor reproduces himself or herself in the mentee. Thereafter he gradually hands over the baton to his once mentee to continue the race. Mentoring therefore gives the mentor the opportunity to pull up the mentee and thereafter hand over to him or her.

One sterling example in my country Nigeria is the legendary Nun; Dr Ann Ward who was an Irish Gynaecologist that came to the then pre-colonial Nigeria in 1959. She was appalled at the poor maternal services at the time with consequent outrageous maternal and perinatal deaths. She settled in the southern area of Nigeria in a village called Anua in the present day Akwa Ibom state. Dr Ward was the pioneer Obstetrician Gynaecologist in St Luke's Hospital Anua (Catholic owned Missionary Hospital). One of the most distressing problems she encountered was the occurrence of the dreaded Vesico-Vaginal Fistula (VVF): a condition from prolonged labour in young women in which there is a connection between the bladder and the birth canal leading to incontinence of urine and faeces. The horrible stigma attached to this condition was terrible and often took away the woman's dignity and self worth. On meeting this hopeless situation, Dr Ward was filled with compassion and worked extremely hard to repair these fistulae thereby giving the women back their dignity and life. She eventually developed a simplified surgical repair procedure which she coupled with intense care in pre-operative preparation and post-operative care. She repaired more than 2,000 of these obstetric fistulae and other devastating pelvic injuries herself, working late into the night under primitive conditions. She also set up periodic "camps" where many more young women were operated on by fellow Obstetricians who flew in from Europe at her request. These visiting Specialists however learnt from Dr Ward's improved procedures which spread across other localities and other countries.

Over the years, Dr Ward started training Nigerian Doctors and Nurses to optimize their knowledge and skills in Obstetrics and Gynaecology. Some of these Doctors were sent to hospitals in the UK for further training. Dr Ward retired due to her failing health in 2006 after serving for almost 50 years in rural Nigeria. She later died in 2015 at the age of 87 years. Today, there is a remarkable improvement of maternal services with marked reduction in maternal and perinatal death. More importantly, there are many skilled and properly trained Obstetricians who have continued the improved maternal care and the repair of obstetric fistulae she was passionate about. It stands to reason that a good number of Obstetricians from Akwa Ibom State and to some extent the neighbouring Cross River State of Nigeria were inspired and motivated either directly or indirectly by Dr Ann Ward. Therefore her legacy of excellent maternal services and skills in repair of obstetric fistulae lives on in these Obstetricians and nurses. In essence, *Dr Ann Ward handed over the baton.*

This is mentoring at its best; grooming men to their very best and handing over to them thereafter.

The deficiency of this crucial step of handing over the baton has led to the failure of many medical training and practices where the expert retires without a replacement.

Handing over therefore is one of the main benefits of Mentorship amongst many others. This is particularly important in the Medical Profession since the medical practice is a type of apprenticeship.

CHAPTER 2

TYPES OF MENTORING

"One good mentor can be more informative than college education and more valuable than a decade's income".

Sean Stephenson

There are many different types of mentoring.
However, most authorities agree that there are basically two types of Mentoring:
- Informal
- Formal

Informal Mentoring
Informal Mentoring is also called *Natural Mentoring*. This type of mentoring process does not involve a structured recruitment, mentor training or matching services. This is the common mentoring type all of us have experienced. Most of this natural mentoring came from our parents, teachers, older siblings and friends; particularly practiced in the traditional African family. Certain knowledge like oral history, skills like cooking, trading, gardening and cleaning are gradually transmitted to the growing child informally. In fact in the African extended family system, each member of the family (grandparents, uncles, aunties, cousin and all) is responsible for each other. These all participate in the upbringing, teaching, training and correction of the growing child. Further correction comes from the teachers, neighbours and family friends. There is therefore a large network of mentors to guide and train the child albeit informally.

Professionally too there are informal mentors which were not chosen from a structured Mentoring programme. These mentoring relationships develop naturally when a senior or more experienced individual meets a younger or junior colleague and both of them strike up a rapport. This type of Mentoring has been well practiced in different professions and settings in the world including in the Medical Profession and Academics.

There are some well recognized significant mentoring systems all in the world. The one type that most of us are conversant with was practiced by the Lord Jesus Christ.

The Discipleship System practiced by Rabbinical Judaism and the Christian church

The Discipleship system in the Bible which was instituted by the Lord Jesus Christ and still practiced today in Christendom is a Mentoring system. The Lord walked with his 12 disciples all the time. There were no formal lectures but the Lord regularly taught them with every given opportunity. He taught them his principles and shared many experiences with the disciples. He used every opportunity to impart spiritual and divine principles to those disciples. Much as many Christians understand that there are many more spiritual issues in discipleship, the basic concepts are the same. It involves an informal relationship where the Lord Jesus Christ himself (obviously of superior knowledge) transmitted knowledge, beliefs and passions over a long period of time to his disciples. He frequently used parables in order to illustrate and simplify his teachings. The disciples continued his teachings after his death and resurrection backed by the Holy Spirit. These disciples went ahead and passed on his teachings and their experiences to many other disciples. Today Christianity as a religion is widely practiced and probably has the largest followers in the world.

Significant Mentoring systems in Nigeria

Elders- Youth system
The elder-youth system is practiced in most cultures of the world. It is very much like parenting but more intense. The knowledge passed on includes the cultures and traditions of the land. Most of the history and cultures are passed on by use of oral history, parables and proverbs. Others include leadership skills, administration, and decision making. Over the years, these youths finally grow into men and continue the same process with the younger generation.

The Apprentice System in Skills Acquisition
The apprentice system in acquisition of skills is a very common mentoring system practiced in Nigeria. This is because there are very few formal training institutions for vocational skills. These skills like hair dressing, tailoring catering, decorations are usually passed on in an informal mentoring system. An apprentice is taken to an established artisan to learn the required skills over a period of time which is determined by the trainer. The skilled craftsman takes the apprentice in a step-wise manner until he has concluded the period of tutelage and acquired the needed skills for the trade. Thereafter, the apprentice launches out to establish on his or her own.

The Apprentice trading skills
This apprentice trading skills is well practiced by the Igbo ethnic group. In Nigeria, the Igbo ethnic group is well known for their business acumen and hard work. *The informal mentoring is one their great strengths.* In this system, a young apprentice is taken to an established trader to learn the trade for seven years. The trade may range from clothes, shoes, electrical equipment, building materials and so on. This apprentice learns the trade in step-wise manner from just service (running errands and cleaning the shop) to

taking on few responsibilities till he can get to the major responsibilities. In fact the big merchants have apprentices who are at different stages in learning the business and service. A time comes when these apprentices all but run the shop while the owner just observes and makes occasional inputs and decisions on major transactions. The apprentices are usually not paid but are provided with accommodation and feeding.

The beauty of this system is that after the stipulated seven years by which time the apprentice must have learnt every aspect of the trade while serving, the master is required to set him up in his own trade. This requires a major financial commitment from the master because the person had not been paid for the services he rendered while serving all these years. This then looks like the full payment for all the services rendered with an added compound interest. Hence the master pays for a shop (usually 2 year rent), fill the shop with goods as well as give him a cash infusion. The trainer merchant/trader is also required to oversee his apprentice in the newly established business till he is able to stand on his own.

Interestingly, once the apprentice is fully established some years later, he picks his own apprentice and the whole process is repeated. This makes the Igbo shops grow in their leaps and bounds seeing that these shops are established in a geometric progression leading to an exponential growth. In every city in Nigeria, Igbos own the most established shops and actually create rivers in the desert. *This success can be credited to determination, hard work and this informal mentoring system.* A popular saying in Nigeria is "Any city without an Igbo man spells doom because survival is impossible in such a city". This captures the determination and sheer will power used by the Igbo man to set up a successful enterprise in any strange land despite all odds.

The Mallam- Almajiri system

The Mallam-Almajiri system is another time honoured Mentoring system amongst the northern Muslims in Nigeria. Mallam means teacher while Almajiri means student hence it is a teacher-student relationship. The Mallam is a renowned Islamic cleric who is versed in the ways of the Islamic prophet. Young boys are taken from their parents to live with a particular Mallam usually in a far location. The Mallam spends time to train them in the ways of Prophet Mohammed. He also teaches them to recite the Koran and all the beliefs and tenets of Islam. On completion, the Almajiris are released back to the society while a new cohort of young boys will be brought to the Mallam for training.

Formal Mentoring

Formal Mentoring is also called *Planned Mentoring*. This type of Mentoring is characterized by a structured program devised in a way where mentors are matched to mentees. This second form of mentoring is becoming more and more popular around the world because the people who have been mentored have given great testimonials. It has therefore become the recommended type of mentoring. Mentors are usually from varied backgrounds. Formal Mentoring can be used in educational, career, personal or venture development. In this formal mentoring, an administrative unit or office in a company or organization, academic institutions, hospitals and companies sets up the relationship between the mentor and the mentee. It is the duty of the administrative unit to solicit and recruit qualified individuals who are willing to mentor. Thereafter, these individuals undergo a training to be better prepared. The unit also matches the mentors and mentees based on their different interests, personalities, qualities and passions. It has been shown that formal mentoring programmes which simply assign mentors to mentees without allowing individuals to make their choice have not performed well. This is because though a mentor and a mentee may seem perfectly matched "on paper", in practice, but may have different working or learning styles. In essence, giving the mentor and the mentee the opportunity to help select who they want to work with is a widely used approach. In fact in most cases, the mentees are permitted to select their mentors based on their perceived needs for example, a young married woman may prefer another married woman who has a rock solid marriage and well brought up children because she is able to understand better the challenges she is facing with juggling family and the hectic Residency Programme together. *Once again, Formal Mentoring is currently advocated as the best form of mentoring in most organizations.*

Other types of Mentoring
These other types are actually considered sub-groups of formal and informal mentorship relationships:

Peer Mentoring
In Peer Mentoring, the mentor and mentee are peers as the name implies. These may be colleagues at the same level, classmates, or trainees in the same programme and at the same stage. However, one person may be more knowledgeable in a certain aspect of the training or another. In some cases, one person may be faster in acquiring the knowledge and skills and as such can provide support and guidance to the others. Being at the same level with similar challenges may make it easier for the colleague to express his or her fears to this peer mentors. One example is that of a House Officer gradually mentoring the new House Officer in the basic requirements and how to organize and circumvent some of the challenges. Peer mentoring

provides a lot of support, empathy and advice considering the fact that both the mentor and mentee are in a similar situation with the same issues and problems.

Situational Mentoring
Situational Mentoring is a short term relationship that arises from a particular situation. It therefore serves a specific purpose. The mentor is usually an expert in a specific topic or skill like social media or internet use. In medicine, it is commonly used in cases of epidemics like in the Lassa and Ebola epidemics in West Africa. Many hospitals and health centers had to invite infectious disease experts to train and mentor their staff on the issues of infection control and universal precautions.

Flash Mentoring
Flash Mentoring is actually a type of Situational Mentoring in which the focus is to receive information for a specific situation. *It is however a one-time meeting between the mentor and mentee.* Flash Mentoring is pertinent when a mentee has a specific defined goal; a goal that scan be achieved in a single forum. The mentee finds a specific mentor to get certain information in order to complete a task. *It places less emphasis on the relationship and more on finding solution amongst a network of people.* The mentee is given a pool of mentors to choose from to help him or her achieve the one-point goal. If there is need for additional assistance, the mentee may request another meeting or reach out to another mentor. *Flash Mentoring is really about convenience.* It is particularly beneficial in job shadowing. Other situations where Flash Mentoring is of benefit include when learning a hard skill, understanding a specific role or on getting an outside point of view particular issue. Flash mentoring is popular for providing a low-pressure mentoring environment that allows the achievement of a short-term objective.

Supervisory Mentoring

Supervisory Mentoring is perhaps the commonest type of mentoring in academic institutions and the Medical Profession. The supervisor is more knowledgeable and is charged with the task of overseeing the junior colleague or trainer. The mentor/supervisor/trainer has the plan, the strategy and directs accordingly. The mentor also acts as the assessor of the mentee. Most of us can relate with this type in academic circles: the supervisor of the academic thesis based on his/her own work in the selected area.

Supervisory mentoring is also seen in the Medical Profession and Residency Programme where the supervisor is the trainer and is also the mentor by virtue of the fact that he is the authority in the mentee's chosen specialty. In view of this, mentor and trainer will be used interchangeably in many instances in this book. *Supervisory mentoring however has the drawback of being a formal mentoring system where the individuals are not allowed to choose themselves.* They were matched by virtue of being in the same unit, department or having similar areas of specialty or research interest. There is therefore a sense of duty to be performed by both parties without the necessary rapport. This can create a conflict of interest in persons who do not have similar ideologies, views or work ethics. I know one such doctor who told her junior colleague. "We are here to do a job. Your job is to do the job while mine is to ensure that you do it well, we do not have to like each other". Such a working relationship was headed to the rocks and it sure got there. Granted, there have been occasions where Residents have chosen their specialties based on the personality and quality of the trainer. Supervisory Mentoring in such a scenario will be much more successful since the mentee chose his or her own mentor and supervisor.

Mentoring Circles
Mentoring can be carried out in circles instead of pairs of mentor-mentee. In mentoring circles, the participants are usually from all levels of the organization who propose a topic. In a mentoring circle, there may be 6-8 individuals who meet regularly with one mentor or two in some cases. They meet regularly once a month or every other month. The duration of the meeting can vary from 1-2 hours. They discuss topics, which motivates them to grow and become more knowledgeable without necessarily looking up to one individual. The topic is generated by the group, the organization or by the contemporary issue on ground. The different mentees go home and think through the topics before the discussion.

This type of mentoring is very useful in scenarios where there are many mentees but few mentors. It has the added advantage of helping the mentees to learn from each other (different skills, approaches, disciplines and methods of learning). More so, in situations where the mentors are two, the mentees also benefit from the knowledge and experience of both mentors. It also opens up the mentees to areas that are not their sole interest and therefore widens their horizon.

One of the challenges of the mentor- mentee pair is the possibility of ill defined boundaries: especially in opposite sex pairs. The mentoring circle has the added advantage of ensuring transparent boundaries since there are many mentees at the same meeting.

A major disadvantage of the mentoring circle is that it does not provide the one-to one personal attention seen in the mentor-mentee pair. The mentor therefore has to learn to mentor many people with individual differences, methods of learning and diverse expectations. Again in some meetings, the issues discussed may not be very important to all the other mentees who may find the topics or issues boring. This may make some mentees disinterested in the meetings while some others may become selfish and repeatedly chose topics that are beneficial to them alone. More so, the scheduling of the meetings will be difficult and challenging because of the number of people involved.

In spite of these disadvantages, the Mentoring circle can be very effective especially where the mentor has been well trained. It is particularly beneficial in the Medical Profession where the expectations of the mentees are basically the same: succeed in their examinations and become successful Specialists. I highly recommend it for medical institutions starting off a formal mentoring programme as well as in situations where the opposite sex mentoring may be misunderstood or misconstrued. In the Medical Profession, mentoring or more appropriately training circles may include programmes like Seminars, Grand Rounds, mortality meetings and Clinic-Pathologic Conferences commonly held in the different departments. It also includes unit presentations which may be much more effective and focused.

CHAPTER 3

BENEFITS OF MENTORING

"Mentoring is a two way tool; the mentor gets wiser while mentoring and the mentee gains knowledge through his or her mentor".

Marisol Gonzalez

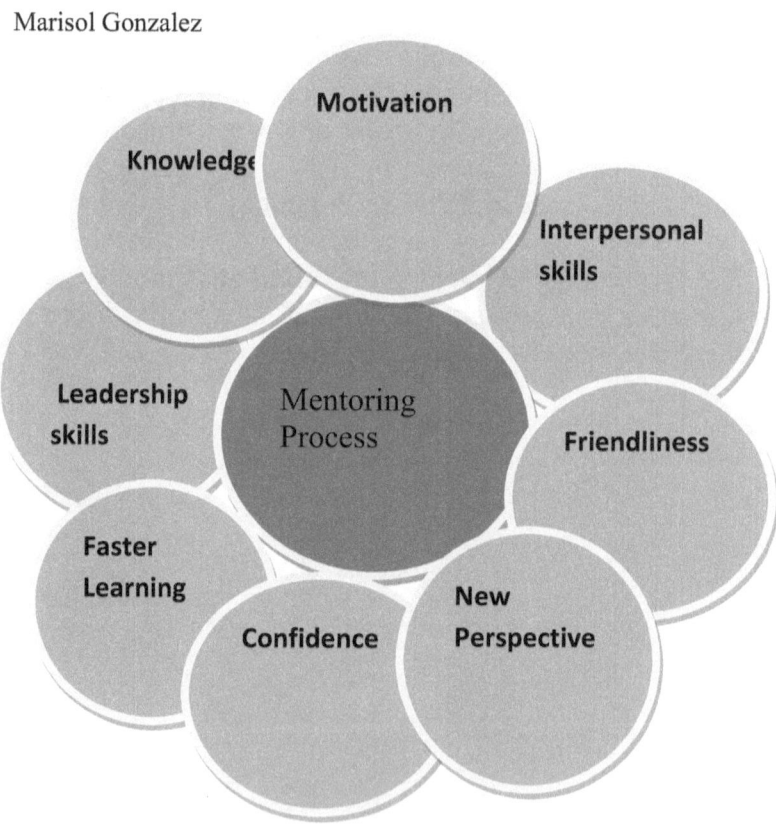

Fig 4. Benefits of Mentoring

The benefits of mentoring are numerous. Some of the core benefits of mentoring for the mentee have been summarized in figure 4 above. However, the benefits will be described in more details as follows;

-Benefits to the mentor
--Benefits to the mentee
---Benefits to the programme manager
----Benefits to the organization.

Benefits to the Mentor

"In learning you will teach and in teaching you will learn"

Phil Collins

There are many benefits for the mentor in the mentoring system. Mentoring is an opportunity for the mentor to give back into the system. The mentor has received much in terms of training, skills though this may have been informal like most of us in the Medical Profession. *Mentoring gives the mentor the opportunity to give back to a mentee and the system, organization or programme.* The mentor is able to share his knowledge, experiences and skills with the mentee.

Mentoring keeps the mentor in touch with current issues and challenges. Medicine is a very fast profession with new ideas, concepts, surgical techniques and treatment guidelines coming out regularly. Mentoring gives the mentor the opportunity to be in touch with all the current concepts and ideas. In mentoring, the mentor is regularly updated by the trainees and mentees especially in the Medical Profession where the trainees are preparing for examinations. I personally learnt the new definition of Stroke from Dr Franklin Dike; a Consultant Neurologist in my hospital during my supervision of his dissertation. It is therefore pertinent for Consultants who are the trainers to attend regularly the post graduate seminars, journal club meetings, mortality meetings and grand rounds. It is within this period that the mentors/trainers learn the current knowledge, facts and concepts from the Residents.

Mentoring *strengthens the mentor's interpersonal relationship skills*. In mentoring, the mentor has the opportunity to relate with different types of junior colleagues over many years thereby helping him to sharpen his relationship skills. His ability to communicate to different mentees is greatly improved as he mentors different people at different times.

Mentoring helps to *re-energize the mentor's career*. The career of a mentor usually receives freshness by virtue of the mentoring process. He may be reminded of his own training and the issues and challenges at the time. He is also able to enhance his own knowledge and skills of not just his specialty but also other related fields. This is especially so when the mentee presents a new challenge. The new challenge spurs the mentor on and helps the mentors to understand challenges in other areas of the health sector.

Mentoring helps the mentor *to develop leadership and management skills*. Management of human resources is one of the challenging aspects of management. Mentoring gives the mentor an opportunity to develop leadership skills especially in the areas of communication. In mentoring, the mentor is required to listen to the views, ideas and the visions of his mentee and carefully guide him to the necessary end point where his potentials are released to realize his goals. It is therefore a practical training in leadership thereby equipping the mentor with fine leadership skills.

Mentoring gives *respect, reverence and credibility to the mentor*. This is because the achievements of the mentee give much credibility to the mentor and the mentoring process. The mentor therefore is boosted by the successes of his mentee since he or she will always be part of the mentee's success. The late Nigerian philanthropist Chief MKO Abiola on giving said; "the hand that gives always stays on top of the one that receives". Mentoring therefore ensures that the mentor remains on top of his career.

Benefits to the mentee

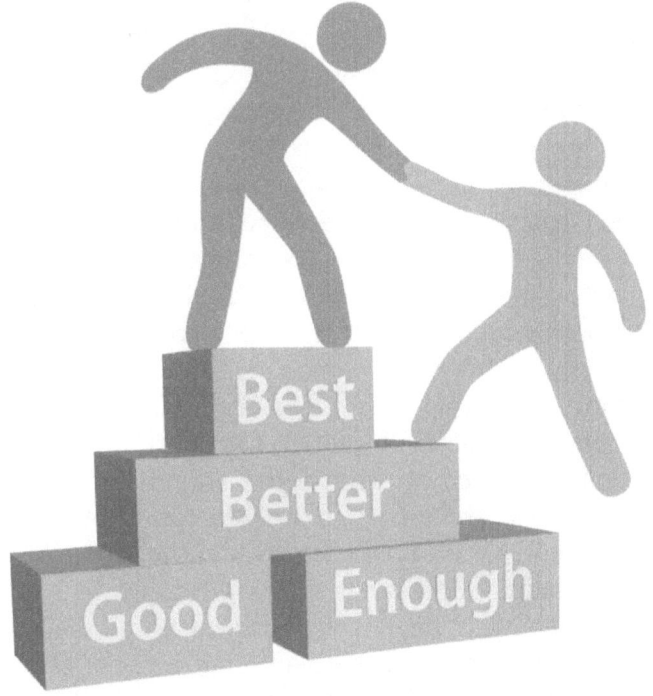

Fig 5: Benefits for the mentee

(Culled from https://www.dreamstime.com)

Most of the benefits of mentoring belong to the mentee because the essence of mentoring is actually to enhance the personal and professional development of the mentee. The mentee's career as illustrated in fig 5 above ascends from **Good** and **Enough** to **Better** and eventually **Best** with the helping hand of the mentor. Some of the well recognized benefits are as follows:

Mentoring increases the mentee's *self-confidence and boosts his morale.* During the process of mentoring, the mentee grows more confident such that he is able to take better control of his or her career. The success may even be beyond the expectations or the original desires of the mentee. This happened in my own situation. I am an author toady because I had mentors who believed in my ability to write; an ability I hadn't really appreciated in myself. However, these mentors recognized the ability and constantly encouraged me to write. This particular book actually stems from one such person. Dr Mfon Edyang-Ekpa a senior colleague who has been a Medical Doctor/Community Health Physician for more than 35 years and such had been a mentor and still is to many young doctors. She heard me speak on Mentoring on two occasions. Thereafter she called me and told me to write a book on Mentorship. She said that many people had to learn the little that I had shared in those meetings where each lecture actually lasted less than an hour. Her belief in me gave me the needed self-confidence to write this book on "Mentorship in Medicine".

Mentoring *teaches the mentee how to share his ideas and innovations.* In mentoring the mentee has to share his own ideas with the mentor. When his ideas are approved by a person senior and more knowledgeable, he is encouraged to be more innovative

Mentoring *educates the mentee*. Mentoring is also an education and learning process albeit informally. The mentee therefore acquires so much knowledge and skills within the period. Some of these will eventually come in handy in some other scenarios years later.

Mentoring *empowers the mentee with leadership skills*. Leadership qualities and positive attitudes are imbibed gradually from the mentor because it is generally agreed that "Actions speak louder than words". The mentee through relating with the mentor learns how to confront issues during difficult times. "He is a chip off the block" is a common comment that arises from the obvious qualities of the mentor replicated in the mentee.

Mentoring *improves the mentee's interpersonal relationship skills*. Mentoring remarkably improves the mentee's skills in relating with people. He learns how to speak up and be heard since in most cases, the mentor is older and also senior to him or her. This is especially so when the mentee has had the opportunity of having many mentors. All the mentors will have different characteristics and have their individual differences. The mentee will therefore learn from different types of people who present different types of challenges which will enable the mentee to acquire the fine art of human relationship.

Mentoring *provides an important networking contact for the mentee*. The mentor provides and opens up his or her own networking contact to the mentee. These contacts are usually beneficial in many ways.

In Medicine, these may include the following:
Collaboration with studies,
Invitation to conferences and workshops both national and international,
Procurement of much needed medical equipment

Benefits to the Mentoring Programme Manager

In the formal mentoring programme, the programme strengthens the administration abilities of the programme manager. Ideally the manager should be someone who understands the institution or department properly. In a medical training programme, a Consultant is appointed as the Head of Residency Training in the department. Such a person who has worked with the different trainers/mentors and the Residents will make a good programme manager for the department. This is because he understands their individual needs and personalities.

The programme therefore provides the opportunity for the programme manager to practice his managerial and leadership abilities. It also helps the programme manager to practice interpersonal skills as he works with many different types of individuals.

The programme manager is also able to understand the needs of the Residents at different stages in their career.

Benefits to the Organization

The implementation of a mentoring programme in a hospital conveys to all the trainees that the institution is willing in their professional development. Usually the Residents have a heavy work load and may feel unappreciated. Taking this step in mentoring the Residents therefore gives the Residents confidence and makes them more loyal to the training institution seeing that the institution genuinely cares about their progress and professional development.

Mentoring gives the institution the opportunity to gradually train future leaders, administrators and mentors to take over the helm of the affair in due time. It also makes the junior faculty members to grow very fast into senior members very quickly.

Finally the mentoring programme creates *a more positive and enjoyable working environment.* The working environment is charged with enthusiasm since everybody is working towards the same vision: optimal quality and care. The Residents are happy because they realize that people wants them to succeed. They are confident that they can discuss their problems easily and get constructive criticism when there is need. More so, all the people involved are able to relate better hence reducing the interpersonal squabbles. The whole working environment becomes enjoyable like a family.

CHAPTER 4

MEDICAL TRAINING IN NIGERIA

"Regardless of our title and years of experience, we can learn from each other, through mentoring and by being open to learn, we can reach our ultimate potential".

Lily Benjamin

Medical education in Nigeria started formally with the establishment of the Premier Medical School in University College Ibadan in 1948. The curriculum of University College London was adapted with slight modifications to stress Tropical Medicine and emphasis on Paediatrics. Shortly after, four other schools in Lagos, Zaria, Nsukka and Ile –Ife were established.

The initial objectives of setting up of medical education in Nigeria include:
--To provide a sound scientific and professional basis for the training of doctors capable of working anywhere in the country
---To provide training to equip these trained health personnel to render primary health care (PHC)
----To train more community-based doctors
-----To produce doctors who would satisfy internationally recognized standards.

It was expected that the trained doctors would undertake further training towards specialization anywhere in the world. In addition, the system was required to produce Doctors with sufficient management ability to play a leadership role in health care delivery. Seventy years later, these objectives are being fulfilled by more than 40 established medical schools in Nigeria.

Residency is a stage of Graduate Medical Training: a Resident is a medical doctor (one who holds the degree of M.D., D.O., MB, BS, MB, BCh or BM, BCh) who practices medicine usually in a hospital or clinic under the direct or indirect supervision of an attending physician or Consultants (in commonwealth countries). The residency training programme is structured to give in-depth training within a specific branch of Medicine. It is also called Specialist training in some countries. It gradually evolved in the late 19th century from brief and informal programmes for extra training in a special area of interest. The first formal residency programmes were established by Sir William Osler and William Stewart Halsted at the Johns Hopkins Hospital in the United States. The programme later became formalized and institutionalized for the principal specialties in the early 20th century. For many decades, residency was not considered necessary for general practice and only a minority of doctors participated in the training. This was especially so in the developing countries like Nigeria.

The Residency Training Program in Nigeria was formally established in 1974, with the following objectives;

--Providing Specialist Training at a high level and appropriate to the needs of Nigerian population
--To halt the brain drain taking place as a result of relocation of the much-needed medical Specialists to the developed world.

The Nigerian Residency Programme is guided by the National Postgraduate Medical College of Nigeria and/or the West African Postgraduate Medical College making these two colleges the main regulatory and training institutions.

In Nigeria, the residency training is a very hectic programme. The Residents acquire the much needed knowledge usually by rote memorization. Clinical training and skills acquisition take place in the clinical areas viz: ward bed side teachings, teaching in clinics, theatres and laboratories. Didactic lectures which have been the main way of passing on knowledge during undergraduate medical education are generally not used conventionally in residency training. Such lectures are mostly given during the update and revision courses organized by the National Postgraduate Medical College of Nigeria and/or the West African Postgraduate Medical College. Other avenues for acquisition of knowledge and skills are the presentation of seminars, grand rounds, conferences and workshops.

Consultants are appointed and authorized to act as leaders, teachers, role models and mentors charged with guidance of the Residents and House Officers who are the trainees and mentees. More often than not, the excruciating work load is such that the brunt of the work falls mostly on these Residents. This makes the training tough considering the sheer vastness of the knowledge the Residents are expected to acquire with this type of workload. Nigeria has many Residency Programmes domiciled in different teaching and Specialist hospitals in the country which produce more Specialist than most other African countries.

The Nigerian Residency Programme is geared towards producing Specialists in different specialties to render expert care for different conditions in Nigeria. All the programmes are medical and dental. The basic entry qualification into the programme is MMBS, MBBCh or BDS. The programme is structured to train experts that are versed in management of diseases in Nigeria but of best practice standards who can put up their shoulder anywhere in the world.

There are two bodies that govern Specialist training in Nigeria as earlier mentioned: the West African College of Physicians and the National Post Graduate Medical College of Nigeria. These two colleges develop and organize the curricula for professional postgraduate education in the various specialized branches of Medicine and Dentistry. They also oversee the conduct of professional postgraduate examination of candidates to certify the successful candidates as Specialists. These Specialists are then appointed Consultants in Tertiary Health Institutions and Lecturers in the University Medical and Dental Schools.

The residency training programme is divided into junior residency that takes the first three years and the later three or four years for the senior residency. In all, most of the programmes are completed within five to seven (5-7) years. Few specialties like neurosurgery usually require more time. This depends on how quickly the Resident can succeed in his or her examinations.

There are three stages of the examinations within the programme. The first is the "Primary" examination which most young doctors take after their compulsory year of internship. Most training institutions require that the applicant must have been successful in the Primary examination of the Post graduate medical colleges or its equivalence. The new Resident is referred to as a Registrar. The Registrar is the most junior of the Residents. He/she spends about three year to complete the needed rotations where he acquires the necessary knowledge and skills. Success in the Part 1 examination is the end point. Thereafter, he or she is promoted to a Senior Registrar.

As a Senior Registrar, the Resident assumes more responsibilities in the management of patients in the next three or four years depending on the department. It is within this period that the Senior Registrar chooses a subspecialty. Others include leadership and managerial skills. The Senior Registrar also carries out a research as part of his part 2 assessment. Achieving success in the Part 2 examinations is the end point at which case such a person becomes a fellow which is the end point of Residency Training. Successful Residency training widens the horizon for the fellow.

Thereafter, the Fellow chooses a career path in either of the following areas:

Academic Medicine

These are the medical doctors who are appointed in the universities as lecturers. The lecturers in the basic medical sciences usually have further degrees in Anatomy, physiology and Biochemistry. The medical doctors in Clinical Sciences however are Consultants in different specialties of Clinical Medicine. They also practice in the University Teaching Hospitals. These doctors are charged with formal teaching of both medical students and Residents.

Clinical Practice

Most medical doctors are involved in Clinical practice. This could be Primary, Secondary or Tertiary care. Consultants are appointed in Secondary and Tertiary care to oversee different units and departments. These are mostly trainers and mentors in the profession; though informal in some cases.

Health Administration

Most doctors take up administrative and management positions while still in Clinical practice. In fact, currently a need to include administration courses in the curriculum of Medical Education to enhance the administrative skills of Doctors who will be involved in Administration and Management. Few others however can earn Advanced Degrees in Health Administration and Management. These Doctors are fully involved in Health Administration, Health Policies and Health Management.

Research

Most medical doctors in Academics are also very much involved in Research. However, there are some others who are totally immersed in Research. These are the doctors who work in Research Laboratories.

Global Health

Global Health is the health of populations in the global context; it has been defined as "the area of study, research and practice that places a priority on improving health and achieving equity in health for all people worldwide. There are any organizations involved in Global Health but the World Health Organization remains the umbrella body.

Multi National Companies

Many multinational companies need medical consultants to head the medical department. Pharmaceutical companies usually need medical consultants to function as medical representatives.

CHAPTER 5

MENTORSHIP IN MEDICINE

"Mentoring is a mutuality that requires more than meeting the right teacher: the teacher must meet the right student"

Parker J Palmer

Mentoring in the Medical Profession in Nigeria is not entirely new having been practiced informally before now especially in the western part of the country. Nigeria is a very diverse country in terms of geography, religion, ethnicity and culture. Though the English language is our lingua franca, there are more than 350 different local languages spoken in the country. However there are three major languages which are Hausa, Yoruba and Igbo: spoken in different parts of the country. Hausa is predominantly spoken in the northern part of the country. Yoruba is spoken in the south western part while Igbo is spoken in the South Eastern part. There is still delta part of the country referred to as "South south". Much as we are all part of the same country, there is so much diversity in the religion, ethnicity, socio-cultural practices and languages. The northern part has more Muslims and a lesser number of Christians. The south however is predominantly Christians with very few Muslims.

As a Medical Doctor in Nigeria, I have had the rare opportunity to practice and observe medical practice and training in these different regions of the country. I was born a Christian in the south Eastern part with my mother tongue being the Igbo Language. In the course of my training, I have trained and or worked in five different Teaching Hospitals in Nigeria in four different geopolitical zones. My experience therefore transverses through the following; two first generation Teaching Hospitals (including the premier Teaching Hospital), two second generation Teaching Hospitals and currently in a third generation Teaching Hospital. I have seen different systems, settings and scenarios in Nigeria in different socio-cultural, ethnic and religious backgrounds. Amidst these diversities, I have been able to appreciate the basic concepts involved in successful medical practice, training and mentoring. In all I learnt that human nature is basically similar and the same basic concepts work irrespective of the geographical location, religious or ethnic backgrounds.

Functions of a Mentor

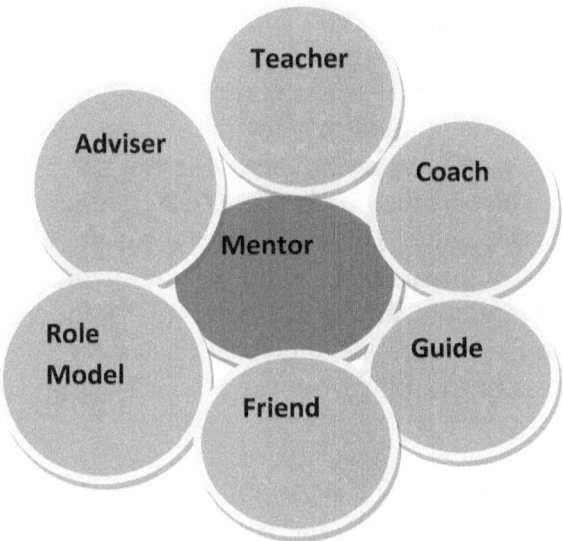

Fig 6. Functions of the Mentor

The cardinal functions of a mentor have been listed in Fig 6 above. The mentor therefore represents all or most of these to the mentee. In all, the mentors are human beings with their different characters and individual differences. However, there are certain qualities that are necessary in order to be a good mentor.

Qualities of the Good Mentors

Knowledge and Expertise

The adage goes *'You cannot give what you do not have or each gives what he has'*. Knowledge and expertise remain the cardinal qualities when choosing a mentor. The reason is obvious; the mentee needs the knowledge, skills or experience for his personal, professional and career development. However, in the Medical Profession there is usually no need to emphasize this fact. This is because, Medicine and Surgery is acknowledged as an extremely difficult course to read. The sheer vastness of knowledge required for a degree in Medicine and Surgery is overwhelming. It presupposes then that anyone who graduates as a medical doctor usually has the required knowledge it takes to be there. Further specialization gives such a person much more expertise especially in his or her area of specialty. The inference is that the knowledge and expertise are usually in place for the medical doctors who are the trainers and mentors. This is the reason that I personally do not lay much emphasis on knowledge and expertise in speaking or writing to medical doctors.

Experience
The mentor in the Medical Profession is preferably one who has experience in the area in which the mentee needs. This is the reason it is important for the mentee to choose the mentor. An aspiring Cardiologist may be better mentored by a senior Cardiologist than an Ophthalmologist since the Cardiologist has had similar experiences and challenges as the young mentee. A trainee Surgeon will need to train under a senior Surgeon to acquire the much needed surgical skills. These experiences count a lot in training and mentoring.

The mentee may also choose a mentor based on the certain similarities in their personal lives. For example, a young married female doctor may fare better with a married female mentor who faced similar challenges with marriage, pregnancies, and nursing babies during residency. She will be more likely to appreciate the struggles of the mentee than a man or single female. Other areas of experience that will guide the mentee in choosing a mentor include experience in research, authorship, management, administration and leadership. The mentee has to choose the area of impact that will enhance him and advance his career and professional development.

Availability
Availability is the most important quality of a mentor in any discipline more so in Medicine. The knowledge, expertise of the mentor is of no use to the mentee if the mentor/trainer is absent. Medicine is a type of apprenticeship and the clinical knowledge and skills especially are only passed to the junior doctors and mentees when the trainer is present. One of the cardinal requirements of mentoring remains the face-to-face communication. Some have modified this face-to-face communication to using chatting or Skype and social media in general. These methods may work in other disciplines but not very well in medicine. *Absenteeism therefore is a No-No in the mentoring process.* The mentor has a wealth of experience that the mentee does not have and must be available to share such for the process to be successful. As they say, 'if your absence does not create a gap and or your presence does not make a difference, then you were irrelevant in the first place". This is because the knowledge, skills leadership and communication skills cannot be transferred in absentia. *An absentee trainer or mentor therefore is irrelevant to the trainees and mentees.* All

mentors and trainers must be available to the mentees and the trainees.

Good Conduct/Examples
The mentor is also a role model and as such should be of good conduct and example. Anytime, any day, actions speak louder than words. Mentoring is a training, an influence and an impartation programme. This means that the lesser is trained of the greater: if that be the case, the mentor commands some respect from the mentor. However, respect is earned and never forced. When the mentor is of poor conduct and a bad example, the usual respect is lost. In such a scenario, there is a breakdown of the entire mentoring process. Mentoring is similar to leadership in many ways. No one can buy into a mentor or leader whom he or she disrespects because of his own poor conduct. Poor conduct and behaviour of some is the reason some people do not believe in mentoring. They can see that the life and practice of the mentor or trainer is contrary to the role model they expect him to be. The negative influence of such mentors and trainers is a huge minus to the whole concept of Mentoring.

Commitment
The mentoring programme is a professional relationship. It takes two to tango. The mentor must be committed to the idea and process of mentoring. Mentoring cannot be forced on a person who has other interests outside mentoring and training. Such a mentor will become an absentee mentor. This is the reason the programme manager has to take time to identify persons who are motivated and interested in mentoring before matching them with mentees.

Capacity and ability to encourage and motivate
The ability and capacity to motivate and encourage are important qualities that the mentor should possess. This is because mentees are human beings. Residency is a double pronged programme as earlier said. The Resident doctor in Nigeria is a full time medical doctor as well as a full time post graduate student. Each aspect of the Residency Programme is hectic. Superimposed on these are the individual's personal challenges with family, ill health and other personal issues. Some medical doctors have chronic diseases like cancer, HIV/AIDs and psychiatric ailments. The current high suicide rate noted amongst medical doctors underscores the fact that medical doctors take of others without taking care of themselves. Hence, the trainee is a young doctor who is encompassed with a huge work load irrespective of what else is happening in his or her personal life. Therefore, the ability to challenge and motivate a doctor going through serious problems while undergoing residency is very important.

In the Nigerian Residency Programme, the Resident undergoes examination, at different stages before being promoted to the next level. Some of the examinations may go awry which is very discouraging to the Resident who had prepared earnestly to be successful in the examinations. The encouragement and motivation of the trainer/mentor is of paramount importance in such a scenario. This encouragement will give the trainee back his or her self confidence and motivate him to succeed in the next examination.

Inspiring
The mentor should have the ability to inspire his mentee for great things. The mentee should be inspired by relating with the mentor. In essence, the mentor should not be dormant in his chosen field; His or her ability to grow and

achieve great things helps the mentee to also attempt to do great things himself. The mentee looks up to mentor and will be inspired to achieve great or greater things than his mentor if he or she is achieving great things. Mentoring therefore energizes the mentor's career when he knows that people are looking up to him or her.

Qualities of the Good mentee

Thirst for Knowledge
The mentee should be someone who is thirsty to acquire knowledge and skills. My favourite illustration is that of pouring water on the ground. When the ground is already wet, the newly poured water will not be absorbed water because the ground is already saturated. In fact the extra water may actually make a mess on the ground and eventually form mud. On pouring water on a dry parched ground however, the water is sapped in a matter of seconds. This dry parched ground also absorbs more and more water. Furthermore, the person pouring the water is more likely to keep pouring on the parched ground seeing that the ground needs the water. This type of scenario is what occurs when a trainee is ready and thirsty to learn. Such trainees ask many challenging questions, they read up topics and are ready to discuss. For those in clinical medicine they clerk patients and are ready and willing to present and discuss the case. They ask questions and are inquisitive. To such Residents, I have had to reply 'I do not know, I will look it up'. Those kinds of mentees and trainees are a delight to teach train. They comprise a challenge to the teacher/ trainer. On the other hand, the ones who think that they already know lose out on further information and training. It is just as the Chinese put it "When the student is ready, the teacher will appear". The teacher is more comfortable with a ready student. The thirst to learn makes the mentee committed and available as the

mentor. It is not easy to mentor an absentee and non committed mentee.

Humility

God resists the proud and gives grace to the humble. The Mentoring process is a training process and as such, the lesser is trained of the greater. The mentee must be humble to learn; *arrogance and training are mutually exclusive.* No teacher can successfully train an arrogant person. I once had a trainer during my residency who was reputed to be a very difficult person by other Residents. I was repeatedly warned to be careful of him. However I underwent the training for one year without any negative incidents. Years later, he repeatedly tells everyone that I was the best Senior Registrar that he ever had. In retrospect, all that I remember is that I was quick to accept my mistake, apologize for them then learn and make amends where possible. This is the reason he rated me so highly. Some of my colleagues who were very intelligent and more knowledgeable than me considered themselves too good and beyond mistakes and rather argued with the Consultant. My own ability to quickly acknowledged my deficiencies and learn were the qualities which impressed this supposedly difficult man and I learnt so much from him because he was a very good Neurologist. Some of my colleagues on the other hand, didn't get much out of him and his great clinical knowledge and skills.

Good conduct

Good conduct is an important quality for both the mentor and mentee. It is always easier to deal with anyone who is well behaved than the badly behaved type. The person with good conduct is more likely to learn because the mentors and trainers find the relationship with him easier. In times of connecting the mentee to positions, the mentor will find it easier to recommend the mentee with good conduct. He will be ready to open up his networking contacts because he is confident of his conduct and character.

Respectful and Responds well to constructive criticism
The ability to respond well to constructive criticism and correction is a very important quality for a mentee or trainee. The trainee or mentee should understand, that as a learner, he or she will make mistakes and this will be criticised by the trainer. Granted, in some instances, some of the trainers may over do it like the Surgeon that throws surgical instruments at his Residents. This is definitely overboard. However, the trainee's response to this trainer's excesses will make the difference between a failed or successful training programme. In as much as the trainers should not run the Residents down or go overboard, the Residents themselves should develop a respectful demeanour that makes them to respond well to criticism.

A respectful Resident or House Officer is a delight for any Consultant. On one occasion, I sent a student out of the class for inattention while I was teaching. He had been busy preparing a seminar that was unrelated to the topic I was teaching. The student waited outside for me to finish the lecture just to apologise his for his wrong conduct. That student's wonderful response impressed me immensely and I have never forgotten him; I would be willing to recommend him if need be because he is respectful. A mentee or trainee who is argumentative, incorrigible and difficult to teach is discouraging and disheartening to mentor and trainer.

CHAPTER 6

TYPES OF MENTORS

"It's good to have female or minority role models. But the most important thing is to have mentors who care about you and they come in all colours".

Condoleezza Rice

Mentors are human beings with individual styles and personality. Often times, medical students or Residents may prefer one Consultant's approach to another. I usually tell them that medicine is too large to be taught in one particular manner and the teachers are persons with individual differences. They should therefore adapt to each teachers style and learn what they can from their different Consultants. However, there are some recognized types of trainers and mentors whose inputs make a remarkable positive or in some case a negative impact on the trainee or mentee. These will be discussed as good and bad mentors.

Types of Good Mentors

Good mentors and trainers come in different shapes. They have their individual differences and are different inputs in their mentees /trainees.

The types of good mentors are described as follows:

The Challenger

The Challengers are not always popular trainers or mentors. This is because they push their mentees too hard and actually overstretch their trainees. They cause their trainees and mentees to hit key milestones and sweat out the details. The Challengers are hard workers themselves and insist on same for their mentees and trainers.

The surgery department Jos University Teaching Hospital (JUTH) in Nigeria from the years 2003 to 2009 typifies my best example of the Challengers. Residency training in Nigeria is difficult as earlier noted. The surgical postings are particularly hampered by poor infrastructure. The JUTH department of surgery however made it work and trained many sterling Surgeons by challenging their trainees and mentees. The trainers stretched the Residents who spent unending hours inside the theatre. The Residents had to read and reread their textbook of operative surgery in order to have the procedure at finger tips before they were allowed to participate in the surgery. Some of the Residents slept in the hospitals on nights they were not on call just to meet up with the demands placed on them by their Consultants. Their post graduate seminars were especially tough sessions. The whole department sat to listen while one the Registrar was presenting a topic. Thereafter, he or she would entertain questions from all the Consultants for almost an hour. The trainers were critical and some of these questions were asked in a harsh manner such that in most cases, the young Doctor will burst into tears. The sessions were particularly hard-hitting. In view of this, the Registrar scheduled for the next week will study harder to surpass his previous colleague and also avoid being upset. Once again, the scenario will be repeated again because the Consultants came out with even tougher questions every week.

This style of training may not go down well with the developed world who frowns on criticism and discouragements as instruments of training. However, what was the resultant effect of this kind of training? *The surgery Residents became phenomenal.* All of them became extremely good such that they had a whooping success rate of approximately 100% in each examination (more 50% of the total success in the West African College of Surgery Examination). All Consultants who had their training in

West Africa will agree with me that this high percentage is a remarkable feat. The JUTH Surgery department became designated as the best centre for the training of Surgeons in West Africa within the period. This was because the trainers were Challengers who raised the bar very high. The Residents rose up to meet the bar and all became exceptional by meeting the challenge of their trainers and mentors. The Challengers make good trainees and mentors because they bring out the best in their trainees if the mentees/trainees are willing to take up the challenges.

In another scenario (in another Teaching Hospital), a Resident was asked by the Consultant in Surgery to copy the whole chapter on 'Pre-Op care' as a punishment. This particular Resident refused to undertake the punishment which he thought was unrealistic and irrelevant. Much as this punishment was overboard, it would have given that Resident the opportunity to read that whole chapter with consequent acquisition of a very good knowledge of pre-op care which will be relevant to him some day. This therefore was a "*challenge*". It looks to me that this Resident missed a great opportunity to have distinguished himself.

The Challengers are usually not popular as noted earlier because they are slave-drivers and hard task masters. They overwork and overstretch their trainees and mentees. They give impossible deadlines. Their assignments, punishments and expectations are within the Herculean range. They push their mentees beyond that which most will consider reasonable, realistic or even relevant. In so doing however, they mould their mentees into the best possible form; they bring out the best in them.

The Cheerleader

The Cheerleader is a great supporter and gives the mentee the needed confidence to achieve great things. Most of us have cheer leaders from our parents, spouses, classmates and good friends who love and believe in us. Much as they love us, they may not fully understand the nitty-gritty and challenges involved in the hectic Medical Profession. Therefore, having a senior colleague in the profession as Cheerleader who understands the challenges and what it entails to succeed in the programme is a tremendous asset. The Cheerleader is genuinely happy for the success of the mentee but will also cheer the struggling mentee. *Note that the Cheerleader is not a flatterer.* He is someone who can make a sincere honest assessment and sees the potentials that the mentee may not be aware. I have been a medical practitioner with most of my passion immersed in clinical practice and training. However, my being an author today is because I had Cheerleaders (outside my family and friends) who encouraged and boosted my confidence in writing. Of particular mention is Udeme Ekrikpo (Consultant Nephrologist): a dear colleague in the same hospital was the first person to see the book that I was writing and exclaimed that it was a good idea. His response gave me the much needed confidence. There have been others like Dr Victor Umoh, and Dr Sylvia Akpan (Jnr) who regularly cheered me on. This particular book on Mentoring was the idea of another Cheerleader: Dr Mfon Edyang-Ekpa who encouraged me to convert the talks that I had given on "Mentoring in Medicine" into a book. This is the mark of Cheerleaders. They see the potentials that the mentee may not have appreciated in themselves and cheer the person. Their belief and echoes of "You can do it" gives the mentee the confidence to achieve great things.

The Idea Generator
The Idea Generator is the mentee's "Thought Partner". They open up the mentees thought processes and send them thinking. The Idea Generators are the ones that unlock the mind of the mentee giving him or her great ideas which lead the person to uncharted areas of new experiences and new opportunities. I am an author today because Dr Kingsley Mayowa Okunoda (Consultant Psychiatrist; Jos University Teaching Hospital) asked me write books to make Neurology easier. He is my idea generator. In addition, Dr Victor Umoh has graciously acted as my sounding board for many years. He gave me further ideas to enhance my authorship of more books. He sent me thinking of all other possibilities.

The Educators
The Educators are the teachers who are gifted with the ability to simplify difficult concepts. They take their time to explain the basic principles. They are sought after and it is common to see medical students and Residents gravitating around such for the simplified ways in which they present all the difficult issues. Educators may use frequent stories and parables to illustrate the topic. Lord Jesus was a great teacher and always had a parable to teach his disciples.

During my Residency Programme in Internal Medicine, I was not comfortable with Rheumatology. This was until Prof Olufemi Adelowo (Professor of Rheumatology) gave us a scheduled lecture in the Part 1 Update course in Lagos, Nigeria. He started the lecture with basic definitions of everyday medical words like *arthritis, bursitis, synovitis, tendinits, and rheumatism.* He further explained the difference between monoarthritis, oligoarthritis and polyarthritis. He took time to explain all the basic concepts, reclassified the whole of Rheumatology in a simpler manner. Thereafter he gave us wonderful lectures on

Rheumatoid Arthritis and Systemic Lupus Erythemathosus. By the end of those two hours, all my confusion had been cleared. That was an Educator; they give the basic skeleton leaving the mentee or trainee to attach the muscles with ease. Educators make good trainers and mentors because they take their time to teach and educate.

The Coach

The Coach is the one that walks with the mentee in times of difficulties. A good Coach doesn't solve the problems but is able to help the mentee see the problem and challenges clearly. The Coach observes, listens and asks focused questions. Coaches are able to help the mentee to prioritize all the issues: such that the more important issues are given preeminence in the hierarchy. In this way, the mentee is able to tackle the most important issues on the list first leading to a remarkable achievement. This means the minor issues which do not have much impact may be left behind but there is a huge sense of achievement having solved the bigger issues already. The Coach can also suggest strategies for solving problems and can help the mentee see "bigger picture".

The Librarian

The Librarian is a moving library or an encyclopaedia. They have a wealth of information on almost every issue. The Librarian knows a resource for most needs and is aware of where to go to get questions answered or to get things done. They know the best or easiest text books, the best journals to subscribe for and the best courses or workshops that will benefit the mentee. They know the best methods to acquire that difficult surgical skill or procedure. They know the best websites, grant application, purchase of good but cheap instruments and equipment.

The Librarian is a good mentor to have especially for those looking for jobs, researchers who need literature and other materials. Dr Charles Amanari (a Plastic Surgeon) my friend and colleague is a Librarian. He has information on almost everything and can source for it with ease. Over the years, he has given me so much information and resources that have enhanced my career, professional development and achievements. Dr Amanari was the person who introduced me to both Pay pal and Amazon giving me the immense benefits of a Pay pal account and shopping on Amazon. Other resources he has provided for me over the years include textbooks, questionnaires, journals, reference managers. He also guided the purchase of my current laptop and functional internet access amongst all other information. Thus as a Librarian, he has given me so much information and resources that have advanced me in my personal and professional development despite the fact that we are not in the same specialty.

The Connector
It is said that "it is about whom you know" but *"it is not just about whom you know but also whom you know also knows and whom he is willing to connect you with"*. The Connector is one of the most important mentors a mentee starting off a career needs. The Connector gets satisfaction from making connections between novices and benefactors. They willingly open up their personal or professional network to others. Their support or introduction can go a long way to enhance the mentee. They are motivated by connecting people with one another to share ideas, passion and energy.
The Connectors are persons who have notable or respected accomplishments in their areas of interest. Their word is greatly honoured amongst their peers. They therefore stake their names, reputation and credibility by introducing or recommending an untried quality. Young Residents and Consultants starting off in their career may find it difficult to be recognized in the absence of a Connector. Amongst

Nigerian professionals those from the South West geopolitical zone (Yoruba ethnic group) are noted to have more class, clout, prestige and accolades. This is because of their passion in mentoring albeit informal in most cases. More so, the mentors are very good connectors who introduce their mentees with ease. This enviable quality should be emulated by all other professional in Nigeria.

The Teammate
This is probably the mentor that is mostly like a good friend. The Teammate is an awesome listener where the mentee can sound off all his frustrations and pent off anger. All the Teammate does is just listening. He understands that there is no need for a lecture. The Teammate does not proffer any solutions to the problems nor give a motivational speech to spur on the troubled mentee. Often times, by the time the mentee has sounded off, he may actually be able to see his problem more clearly and go ahead and solve it himself. *Good listeners make good Teammates.* All the Teammate does is to give his time and a listening ear. In the brouhaha of the busy and hectic Residency Programme where many people believe that they have the panacea to all the problems and are ready to dish them out, the Teammate is a huge asset.

In all, there is no person who wholly fits into only one specific type. A truly great mentor often embodies more than one of these personality profiles. It is all about mentoring dexterity which is having a mentor who knows when to push, when to caution or correct. He or she will also know when to teach, when to inspire and when to applaud. Such a person has been referred to as the **"Composite Mentor".**

Again, mentors are human beings too and as such are not perfect beings. They will therefore have one or two Mentoring lapses. In essence, each mentee naturally has his or her unique combination of personality attributes. *In the end, it's about finding the right mentor-mentee combination at the right time that matters most.*

Note:
A new and upcoming trend is having **multiple mentors.** This can be helpful because we can all learn different aspects from each other. Having more than one mentor will widen the knowledge of the person being mentored. These different mentors have different attributes, strengths and qualities. In essence, a Resident from Anaesthesia can pick a Surgeon who is a prolific writer and researcher to mentor him in the area of research.

Types of Poor Mentors

The Absentee Mentor
The Absentee mentor is probably the worst type of mentor to have. Mentoring even when it is informal requires quality time spent between the mentor and mentee. Mentoring and medical training cannot be carried out in absentia no matter the mentor's level of education, knowledge and skills. *The Absentee mentor or trainer is irrelevant to the mentee and trainee.* Some of these are busy bees who have too many fish to fry and the mentee or trainer is not a priority. The mentor must have valuable time to make impact on the mentee. Nothing else can make up for unavailability. *Unavailability is a No-No in Mentoring and training.*

The Naysayer
The Naysayer repeatedly speaks against ideas and habitually expresses contrary opinions. He thinks of all the

reasons that will make a venture might fail, rather than the ways and how it might succeed. *"A good mentor never tramples on big dreams."* The Naysayers are terribly discouraging to the mentee. One of the reason the Naysayers behave they do may be because they never had the idea in their time or even now and therefore resent the idea of a junior person being a pace setter. Some Naysayers honestly do not see good in any novel idea or innovation because they concentrate on obstacles and actually expand them. Naysayers do not look out for or encourage solutions. The person who listens to the Naysayers never makes great achievements. I remember when I started writing my first book, I mentioned it to a very senior respected colleague who discouraged me and told me that writing a book was most unnecessary. He went ahead told me the story of someone who had written a book and detailed all that went wrong with the book. In all honesty, most of the things he said were correct it made me so discouraged that I stopped writing. After a while, I gathered some courage and just plodded on with that first book.

The Naysayers are not good mentors. Their frequent cry of *"It can't be done"* puts a ceiling on the mentee/trainee and prevents such a person from achieving great things. *Avoid the Naysayer if you can or stop your ears.*

The Bloviator

The Bloviator is over bloated by his or her own achievements and does not think that his mentee may achieve anything more than he already has. He is unwilling to listen intently and is quick to wax lyrical about his own war stories and trophies, whether relevant or not. In essence, he inadvertently belittles the mentee and as such does not encourage or boost their mentees. The Bloviator trivializes the concerns, interests and passions of the mentees. In addition, such a person neither shows nor admits any personal weaknesses but rather expects to be the role model in all aspects of career development and personal values. The Bloviator believes that he knows it all. This kind of person who is not willing to accept his or mistake is not a good mentor. The Bloviator can easily lead the mentee astray since he is not able to retrace his steps and reconsider the issues: he knows it all.

The Hoarder
Hoarders are very poor mentors because of their selfishness. Selfishness, in general, is not exactly a great trait for anyone to have, but it's even worse when it's seen in a mentor. A selfish mentor is a bad mentor; plain and simple. Such a person cannot freely give his time, knowledge, experience, ideas, and or feedback. He is unwilling to share either knowledge, skills, experience, websites and their network of contacts or anything that will benefit and enhance the mentee or trainer.

One such was a professor of Histopathology whose retirement was akin to closing down the histopathology laboratory. The tertiary hospital had to send their samples elsewhere while sending the Residents to other Teaching Hospitals for training. The Hoarders defraud not only their mentee or trainees but more importantly, they also defraud the institution, organizations and society at large. Unfortunately, they also defraud themselves of respect, reverence, honour and the accolades that good mentors enjoy. Furthermore, Mentoring as illustrated earlier is handing over the baton. *The Hoarders neither hand over the baton nor do they reproduce.* How sad!

The Puppeteer
The Puppeteer makes the mentee his puppet. He does not guide the mentee or trainee to make his own choices, decisions and career pathway. The Puppeteer will usually insist on his way in all the issues. The projects, researches or thesis worked on will have to be according to his

interests or passions. Such a person is unable to identify the mentees individuality, personality, qualities strengths, passions and interests different from theirs. He expects that every piece of advice he/she hands down should be followed to the letter. He will take offense if an alternate path is taken.

The Puppeteer's method is to create someone that is exactly like him or her ('mini me'). This does not allow the mentee achieve his or her own full potential. The good mentor will observe his mentee and note his strengths, qualities interest or passions and guide him or her appropriately. Collaboration with persons with different strengths makes the organization, hospital and institution richer. According to Benjamin Disraeli, *"The greatest good you can do for another is not just to share your riches but to reveal to him his own."*

I hereby appeal to all mentors and would be mentors ***"Please do not clone yourself".***

Good mentoring is about guiding the mentee to realize his own innate potentials and be the best that he or she can. The best role ever is to "star you"; every person should bloom where he or she is planted. This is the whole essence of mentoring.

When the mentee is able to express his individuality and innate qualities, the specialty or unit as a whole is richer for it. As the pioneer Neurologist in University of Uyo Teaching Hospital in Nigeria, I had a passion to start off the Uyo Stroke registry. This passion knew no fruition for about 7 years. There were always obstacles and road blocks. However, when Dr Franklin Dike was appointed as a Consultant Neurologist, with him overseeing the project, the Uyo Stroke Registry took off within a month. This is the essence of allowing individual expressivity.

I love the way Mother Theresa puts it *"You can do what I cannot do, I can do what you cannot do, together we can do great things"*.

The Compromiser

Mentors are usually role models in many aspects of the profession. The mentees look up to the mentors and trainers in knowledge, skills conduct and character. The Compromiser is not a good role model because he is known to bend rules and use short cuts thereby compromising quality, standards and ethics of the profession. This type of mentor who does not live up to these expectations looses all the respect and reverence of the mentee. As Ralph Waldo Emerson put it *"What you are is so loud that I can hear what you say"*. Some persons have chosen not to be mentored because of having known such persons who do not meet their expectations in terms of conduct and character. Continuing with such a mentor or trainer is dangerous because the mentee or trainee does not acquire high standards of practice, conduct and character.

A different way of compromising is when the mentor or trainer is ready to condone wrong and bend the rules in order to protect the mentee. In some cases, these mentors may be under some influence e.g. political, financial or otherwise. They are driven by fear and as such are unable to take a firm stand on anything wrong making the mentee or trainee untouchable. These types of untouchable mentees become incorrigible and are bad examples for other trainees. Their *untouchable* status gradually disrupts the whole training and mentoring programme causing moral laxity and decadence.

Unfortunately some of the wrongs being covered up eventually blow up with dire consequences. This causes a lot of embarrassment and disrespect to the mentor: he loses credibility with his peer, colleagues and the entire hospital community.

More so, considering that the trainee is a doctor, the Compromiser does a great damage to the society by releasing an incompetent doctor or Specialist to the unsuspecting public. The problem with this is that *'Bad medical practice is like a stone thrown into the market; you will never know who will be hurt"*. The person who will be badly treated by that incompetent doctor may be anybody including the relatives of or Compromiser himself. It is a small world.

The Vulture

The vulture sees mentoring or training primarily as an opportunity to advance his or her personal agenda. The whole process is planned with the outcome already known. Vultures are generally users and devourers. In the Nigerian system where there is not much in terms of research grant and support, most researchers collect their data themselves and also sponsor the research from personal pockets. The Consultant who uses the Residents and House Officers only for the purpose of data collection with no gains for them is regarded as a vulture. He or she does not impact their knowledge or career and professional development in any way.

In some other cases, some consultants may have a research idea that is cost intensive and may give it to his Resident as his Part 2 dissertation. In most of these cases, the cost implications are usually overwhelming for the Resident. This is actually some sort of manipulation.

In some cases, some Consultants just use the Residents to run their private practice which is not part of the residency training programme to the best of my knowledge.

Painfully there are other Vultures who are interested in sexual favours and or some other self-fulfillment schemes. There is usually little or no gain for the mentee. Having vultures in the system is disastrous to the institution because is causes a lot of discouragement to the mentees and trainees from mentoring programme.

CHAPTER 7

THE PROCESS OF MENTORING

"The key to being a good mentor is to help people to become more of who they already are: not to make them more like you".

Suze Ormen

"You don't have to have all the answers; you just have to be willing to share what you know"

Unknown

Four stages have been recognized in the formal mentoring process as represented in the diagram below.

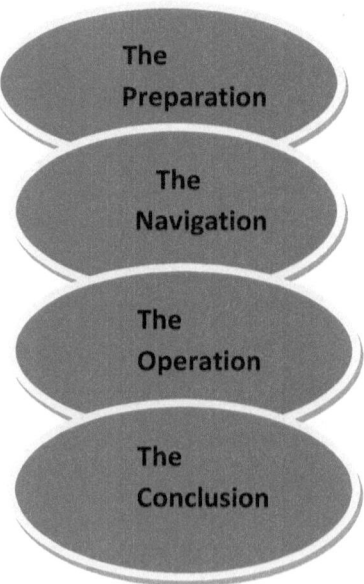

Fig 7: Stages of the Mentoring Process

Phase 1

The Preparation
Components of the preparation stage are as follows: --

-Decision
---Self Assessment
-----Acquaintance and
--------Role Definition

Decision
The preparation starts when the two individuals involved make the decision to be part of the programme. In the Residency Programme, the Consultant makes the decision to be a mentor and trainer to his Residents albeit informally. The Resident as well on being enrolled chooses to be a mentee also knowing that he or she will graduate to become a mentor: peer mentoring initially and full mentoring later on. In the recommended formal mentoring however, the preparation is more formal though there is still an individual decision to be a part of the programme.

Self Assessment
The mentors are to take time to evaluate their personal motivation and their readiness as mentors. They also assess their knowledge, qualities and skills while also identifying their own areas for learning and developments. The mentee also prepares himself or herself. He or she identifies what he intends to achieve from the mentoring process, his individuals strengths and qualities. He also recognizes the learning technique best suited to his or her personality. This period of self assessment and preparation is especially important when the mentor and mentee are not exactly in the same department: those in the same department have similar expectations from the process. One example is a

situation where an obstetrician is to be mentored by an Ophthalmologist (for research, leadership, public speaking, statistics and so on).

Acquaintance

In the formal mentoring programme, there is a time to fix an initial meeting to establish some rapport. The mentor and mentee are introduced as a pair and they get to know each other. Salient questions the mentor must ask the mentee are as follows:

1. What is it that you really want to be and do?
2. What are you doing really well that is helping you get there?
3. What are you not doing well that is preventing you from getting there?
4. What will you do differently tomorrow to meet those challenges?
5. How can I help / where do you need the most help?

Role Definition

In this period of role definition, there has to be a clear establishment of the roles and what the mentor can offer the mentee within the mentoring process. The mentor will have to ask himself some crucial questions like; what do I have to offer this person? "Can I work productively with this individual? Do I honestly feel that I can further this person's learning?" In what ways can I enhance this person's knowledge, skills and medical career? In as much as it is normal to expect some initial chemistry between the mentor and mentee like in most relationships, most authorities believe that the chemistry is overrated: it may come eventually. In the formal mentoring programme, it is within this period that further meetings are scheduled and the endpoints are defined.

Inadequate preparation stage has led to the failure of many mentoring programmes. Note that mentoring process may actually come to a conclusion within this time based on mentor-mentee mismatch. Causes of mismatch may be different priorities and or goals, different learning styles, inability to schedule meetings or the unavailability of the mentor or the mentee for the programme amidst others.

Phase 2:

The Navigation
The Navigation period is the second phase where the mentor-mentee pair commences the process treading carefully.
Components of the Navigation Period are

- Style
---Setting of boundaries
------Define and
--------Agreement

Style
The period of navigation is the period of discussing the possible style and methods that will best suit the Mentoring relationship. The learning goals have been laid down properly in the stage of preparation (Phase 1). During this period, the ground rules are discussed. In fact there is an overlap between phases 1 and 2 since the issues may not all be clearly defined within Phase 1. Some of the issues with methods of learning and even the scheduling of meetings may come out gradually as the relationship develops. For some pairs, they may use this as a period of learning a new style when differing styles is noted. However, as earlier noted, the difference in learning styles may actually be the reason that the process will come to a conclusion.

Setting of Boundaries

Setting of boundaries and limit setting is a very important issue in mentoring. Another major issue will be that of defining confidentiality. It is within this period that trust for one another is established gradually between both parties. Mentoring is a process that may grow into a beautiful relationship; character traits that may hamper the process will be noted at this time. Some persons may chose to change the mentor within this period thereby arriving at an early conclusion (stage 4).

Define

The Navigation Period is also the best time to characterize the modalities of the process. This will include issues like the venue, time and the duration of each meeting (when to meet, what to discuss of the phone). The schedules should take into the individual programmes of the parties into consideration.

Agreement

Some have suggested that there should be a "Mentoring Agreement" which should be documented and endorsed by both parties. Salient areas of agreement include the goal of the process, especially *what the mentee intends to learn and the support needed to learn that*. It also includes the frequency of the meetings, the commitment of both parties, the role of the mentor and the success outcomes.

In my hospital, formal Mentoring is still at its rudimentary stages. For now, the new programme allows the mentees to choose the mentors they want to work with.

Phase 3

The Operation

The Operation Phase is the kennel of the Mentoring process. Ideally all the problems should have been anticipated before now. The programme should commence in earnest with gradual progress as measured by achievement of the goals. Successful completion of the Operation phase may lead to either completion or conclusion. In some cases, the Operation Phase never ends but rather progresses to a beautiful friendship.
Components of the operation stage are

Commitment
In this phase, the mentoring process has commenced with the roles clearly defined and all the boundaries set. Both parties work on commitment to the mentoring process. This is the period for learning and developing. By this time, both parties would have learnt how to communicate openly. The mentor within this period should have learnt to nurture mentee's growth by establishing and maintaining an open climate. They are committed to achieving the goals of the mentee. Gradually some of the goals are being achieved; there may be some losses or misses within the period.

Challenges and Criticism
Having learnt how to communicate effectively, the mentor and trainer would have noted some of the mentee's qualities and strengths. This is the time for the mentor to provide challenges, and constructive criticism. The trainee or mentee meeting the challenge makes him better balanced and equipped to strike out on his own. In the residence training in Nigeria and in fact West Africa as a whole, the end point is usually success at the examinations. This

means that the trainer is ready to progress to the next stage of the training.

Continuous Assessment
The operation phase is also characterized by continuous assessment and reflection on the Mentoring process. Time and again, the mentor and mentee will have to sit down to assess the progress of the mentoring process. Have some of their end points been met?

Confidence
The successful progress of the mentoring process since the mentee would have won some few battles with consequent increasing confidence and a boost of the morale. By this time, both would have realized whether the process is beneficial to both of them or not. The Resident would have succeeded in his examinations and is ready to move on as a clinician, academician or an administration. It is then time to move to Phase 4: Stage of Conclusion.

Phase 4
The Conclusion
Most things that have a beginning also have an end. Mentoring may have an end in some cases whereas there is there is no end in some other cases. This is because the mentoring process may blossom into a beautiful mutually rewarding relationship that continues forever just like the family relationships or good friendships that never have an end. Every one of us has some person or persons like that who has been there for us all our lives. We still fall back on them for advice, guidance, in difficult times and all. In some cases, the mentee becomes the support while the former mentor becomes the supported as occurs in parent – child relationships. An adage in the Nigerian Igbo dialect says *"When parents have successfully trained the child, then the child takes over in training the parents"*.

Mentoring can develop to such relationships where the benefits remain many years. In such cases, there is no phase 4(Conclusion) in Mentoring.

However, there are cases that get to this phase 4 where there is need for conclusion and closure. There are signals that indicate that it is time for closure. This will be when the learning goals have been met and the mentee no longer needs the guidance. In such cases, it is time to celebrate the achieved success. Thereafter, both mentor and mentee can move on. *The conclusion may also be because the mentee may still need another type of mentor for other purposes.* The Mentoring process can also be closed when the relationship is no longer effective. Please note that the phase 4 does not necessarily follow the first three phases. Phase 4 can come in Phase 1 or 2 when it is noted that the two individuals will not be able to work together. The sooner an effective process is closed to find more compatible matches, the better for both mentor and mentee

Training and Support for Mentors
In informal or natural Mentoring, there is no training for the mentor. This is like parenting a child or good long lasting friendships. The learning is mostly informal from what is gleaned from other people's experiences. In recent times however, there are books and trainings in parenting to give some much needed guidelines for parents. In the same vein, mentors can be trained to have an easier navigation; that is the essence of this book in the first place.

Types of Training

Train the Trainers Workshops
In Nigeria, the two post graduate colleges organize some of these: the "Train the Trainers" and management courses and workshops for the Consultants who are the trainers and

mentors as already noted. Mentoring is usually taken as one of the topics amongst other issues. The essence is to give would be mentors some knowledge and the needed guidelines. However, there yet remains a knowledge gap that is yet to be filled as most of the issues are not handled.

Institutional Work shop
The organization, institution or hospital should organize trainings and workshops for mentors. However, the training institutions also need their own specially designed workshops and courses for mentors. These types of workshops should be adapted to the special needs of the mentees and the institution.

Continuing Medical Education
Mentoring can be taught during the continuing medical education programmes organized by different medical associations. My personal journey with studying "Mentorship" started from such a lecture given in a welcome programme organized by the hospital management for the new Residents to the residency training programme. Thereafter, I was invited to other CME programmes to give the lecture because of the response. I recommend "Mentorship" as a CME/CPD Topic on a regular basis.

Open mentoring Courses
There are courses organized on line for all mentors and would be mentors. There is a package for new mentors and another for the more experienced mentors.

Books, Journals and online Resources
Books are always a good source of information. People who are interested in training and mentoring need to read books in order to learn and design their own programme. There are also journals, and on line resources of personal

experiences that will benefit anyone who wants to be a mentor.

Nevertheless, all the knowledge and skills needed for effective Mentoring cannot be taught in workshops. Certain aspects can only be learnt by experience as one starts to mentor as we all know: *practice makes perfect*.

Support for Mentors
Mentors need support and challenge
Mentors also need support and challenge from the organization or institution. Topmost is the training support as described above.

Recognition and Reward for Mentors
The rewards for the mentor cannot be overemphasized as already discussed in the benefits of mentoring. In the informal mentoring, the mentees may go ahead and honour and reward the mentors in their own ways. In few cases, the reward may be incredible: beyond the Mentor's wildest imaginations!

One of such incredible recognitions took place last month when the Liberian President honoured his mentor Arsene Wenger by giving him the highest National honour of his country Liberia at a ceremony held in Monrovia on Friday 24th of August 2018. Wenger was inducted into the country's Order of Distinction and given the title of night Grand Commander of the Humane Order of African Redemption.

President George Weah had been born into poverty and brought up in the slums of Monrovia. He took to football because his parents were too poor to send him to school. He moved to play for Tonerre Yaoundé in Cameroun to take his football to another level. The then Cameroonian Coach Le Roy noticed his skills and convinced his friend Arsene Wenger to sign him. In 1988 Arsene Wenger who was the

Coach of FC Monaco signed George Weah: an unknown black. Weah said theirs was a father –son relationship. Wenger showed him love when racism was at its peak. Wenger believed in him saying that he had the talent to be one of the best players in the world. Weah kept on and went on to play for some other prestigious clubs in Europe viz Paris SAINT Germaine, AC Milan and Chelsea. In 1995 Weah won European footballer of the year and World footballer of the year; he remains the only African player to win these awards. His prowess and achievements in the game of football gave him popularity in his country. He went back to school to get the education that eluded him while young. In December 2017, George Weah won the presidential election making him the 52nd President of Liberia. George Weah has lived a very fulfilling life because Arsene Wenger believed in him. In fact, Wenger was the destiny helper that enabled him to become the brand "George Weah" that he is today.

Thirty years later President George Weah remembered the man who opened the career door to him. *He honoured his mentor with the highest honour in his country.* This is how great the appreciation, recognition and reward for a mentor can be. Granted, this kind of honour does not happen every day, but good mentees find ways of appreciating and honouring their mentors.

In the formal mentoring system the mentors in the organization or institution should also be given some sort of recognition for job well done. In every work, there should be a day of reward. This spurs other people on to take on Mentoring.

Suggested ways of Recognition

Awards programme

Most organizations and institutions have designated days to recognize and reward high performers in different areas. This also happens in the hospitals starting from the individual departments. In such programmes, the mentors should be recognized and also honoured.

Thank you mentor day

There may also be a day for just mentors to be recognized and honoured. Such mentors may be nominated by their different mentees. A panel will select the best mentors for the awards. Such a day will be used to honour the best mentor or mentors for the year. Gifts and plaques will be presented to the deserving mentors.

CHAPTER 8

CHALLENGES IN MENTORING

"Leaders should influence others in such a way that it builds people up, encourages and educates them so they can duplicate this attitude in others."

Bob Goshen

Infrequent Meetings

Despite the commitment, there is always difficulty in meeting as frequently required or scheduled. Regular scheduled meetings are part and parcel of formal Mentoring. Most of these arise from the work load of the mentors and mentees. The mentor is a Consultant with his clinical itinerary (clinics, ward rounds, labour ward, theatre sessions and all). He or she is also a Lecturer who has lectures with Medical Students, bedside teaching for students, House Officers and Residents. He is also involved in research, writing of papers or text books and supervision of some other projects. In addition, he or she may have an administrative position with the hospital or university. All these are irrespective of his or her commitments to his or her family, the church or some social life. The same goes for the Resident or House Officer who has similar work load; logging a hectic medical practice with post graduate studies. The post graduate Medical education is spiced with updates and examinations located in another part of the country. Having regular scheduled meeting is tough call. However, failing to meet as scheduled or frequent postponements will quickly erode the foundation of your relationship.

One way of overcoming the irregular meetings is by viewing the meeting as one of the compulsory sessions (lectures, seminar, grand rounds etc) the pair needs to participate in for eventual success. *Mentoring should never be treated as an extracurricular activity.* Both parties should make the Mentoring meetings a priority. Another way is for both parties to prioritize and reduce some of their work load. It is also wise for the mentor to have only one or two mentees at a time. Furthermore, it is important to have mentors and mentees who are very motivated to participate in the programme. Those who are motivated are more likely to make out time for the mentoring programme.

Unrealistic Expectations

The Mentoring relationship is easily wrecked by unrealistic expectations. Once again, this could be on both sides. In the Nigerian Residency Programme, progression comes with success in the stipulated examinations. Some of the mentors and trainers are also examiners. The mentee may expect to scale through the examinations by virtue of having his or her mentor as one of the examiners. This is unreasonable under the circumstances.

Again, some mentees expect that their wrong doings should not be punished especially if their mentor is on the panel. In fact there have been such cases where some misdemeanours were not punished because the trainer or mentor bent some rules. This is actually *'godfatherism'* not Mentoring. In scenarios where the mentor stood his ground to condemn the wrong doing, he is considered uncaring or wicked.

Another unrealistic expectation by the mentee is expecting the mentor to open up his network as soon as the Mentoring process commences. This causes some friction because the mentee may view the mentor as selfish. The mentee should realise that he must prove himself and earn the trust and respect of the mentor before he can be introduced to the mentor's network. Remember that the Connector stakes his name, reputation and credibility on the mentee (an unknown quality). Such a person whom he stakes his reputation on should be deserving and commendable. In essence, earning the trust and confidence of the mentor is what makes him to open up his network and connect the mentee. The mentee has to work hard as well as also wait patiently because this will take some time.

On the side of the mentor, it may be unrealistic for the mentor to overload the mentee with assignments causing friction. As noted earlier, some trainers and mentors are Challengers who push the mentee to work hard. If the trainee or mentee is able to meet the challenge, he excels and distinguishes himself. However, a common pit fall is for the mentor to keep comparing the new mentee or trainee to the previous one who could rise to challenges. In a lot of cases, this may be demeaning and create friction. This is the essence of Phase 1 where the two individuals get to know each other such that the mentor will get to know how the mentee reasons and learns.

Occasionally, a mentor may expect the mentee to accept everything he or she has to offer instead of letting the mentor find his or her own path. Furthermore the mentor may expect the mentee to do all things exactly like him thereby becoming his clone. Such mentors are puppets and do not make good mentors. The mentor is supposed to aid the mentee to realize his own God given potentials. These unrealistic expectations can have a negative impact on the Mentoring relationship.

One way of overcoming these unrealistic expectations is to get to know each other party pretty well during the first stage of the process. The second is to set Mentoring objectives and goals ab initio. This way, there is an agreement as regarding the expectations of the process. Finally, when it doubt or if you're encountering resistance or resentment on the other side it is wise to consult the programme manager.

Overdependence

Overdependence is one challenge of the mentoring relationships. In this situation, a mentor may come to rely on the mentee rather than focussing on the mentees needs. Some of such mentors and trainers may leave most of their own work for the mentee. This is wrong and in fact fraud considering that the trainer is been paid for that job.

Some lecturers have gained promotion by relying on the dissertations, thesis and studies carried out by their mentees, trainees and graduate students. There are situations where this has caused a lot of murmuring and of course disrespect for the mentor or trainer. In some cases, the mentor may project the ideas or work of the mentee or trainees as his or hers thereby getting all the credit from the work. Mentors who are overly dependent on their mentees do not show much interest in the needs of the mentee. Several of these kinds have also been known to lean on the mentee for emotional support.

Likewise, a mentee may also rely too heavily on the mentor's approval and guidance. Much as mentoring provides much needed guidance, good mentoring should enhance growth, confidence and independence. A mentee or trainee who must check in with the mentor before making decisions out of fear of making a mistake or receiving criticism is overly dependent. The essence of Mentoring is to groom the mentee to stand and strike out on his own. During the mentoring process, the mentee should gradually move toward independence. This is not to say that the mentee should become arrogant and disrespectful. The mentees movement towards independence and taking his decisions should be done with decorum. In essence it should be like a gradual weaning off process off the mentor. In order to overcome this overdependence, the mentors should regularly examine their own actions and motives and ensure that they are not being selfish. The mentor should learn to give his mentee and trainee due credit and not rob him of it. This ability to appreciate the mentee's ideas and give him due credit also gives much credibility and admiration and respect to the mentor. A good check for the mentor is to constantly remind himself or herself that the mentoring process is about the mentee and not him the mentor.

In addition, the mentors should learn to gradually wean off the mentees in due time. They should allow the mentees to think for themselves and "grow up". No parent wants a child who is a perpetual baby. The growth is in stages until the child becomes a full-fledged adult who is capable of independent living outside his parent's home and guidance. Achieving such independence for the mentee should also be the desire of the mentor.

The mentees on the other hand need to remind themselves that the mentoring process is a period of learning and growth and that the mentor is actually a source of support, guidance and feedback. They need to make their own decisions. This however should be done respectfully.

Ill Defined Boundaries

Mentoring requires professional boundaries and setting of limits. It is not an opportunity to pry into the mentees personal or private life. In some cases, the mentee may chose to discuss issues in their private or personal lives with the mentor. This usually comes when the mentor has gained the mentees trust. One unethical way of breaking the professional boundary required in Mentorship is by having a sexual relationship with the mentee. Some of the mentors or trainers may even victimize the mentee for refusing the sexual favour. In such a scenario, the mentee may succumb to their demands from the fear of victimization by the mentor. This is very wrong and generally unacceptable because it is an abuse of the programme by the mentor. In addition, it also breaks the professional ethics.

One way of avoiding this is to ensure that the boundaries of the mentoring process are clearly defined *ab initio* during the Phase 1 of the programme. Some have suggested same sex mentoring pairs to avoid sexual insinuations or relationships. This may not always be feasible in some medical specialties where there are not many female mentors. Moreover, in most cases, the mentor-mentee pairs usually stem from the fact that both of them are in the same specialty and as such the matching is unavoidable.

One good way of avoiding the ill defined boundary is to have mentoring circles where there are other mentees always present during the meetings. The prescence of other persons in the circle is protective for both the mentor and the mentee. Mentoring circles however lack the one on one relationship and personalized touch which is valuable in the mentoring pair. Clear definition of boundaries at the beginning of the relationship therefore remains the key in cases of mentoring pair.

Manipulation

Manipulation is common in all human relationships. It can therefore be seen in mentoring relationships practiced by either the mentor or mentee. Once again, the trainer/mentor may ask a mentee to complete the mentor's work under the guise that the mentee will learn better if the mentee actually does the task. It is true that the mentee or trainee will definitely improve his skills because practice makes perfect. However, there is a huge difference between learning a skill and doing someone else's work. It is therefore wrong of the mentor to manipulate the mentee or trainee into doing his or her work.

Another type of manipulation is when a trainer burdens his trainee with the task of carrying out a capital intensive study under the pretext of teaching him or her to carry out quality world-class research. Such a trainee may be overwhelmed with the expensive cost of the study but is unable to complain for fear of victimization. This is a type of an extremely unfair manipulation.

Mentees, on the other hand, may blame their wrong actions or decisions on their mentor instead of assuming personal responsibility. This creates a lot of problems if such a statement is made within a context that pits the programme manager against the mentor in formal mentoring programmes. This again is inappropriate and disrespectful on the part of the mentee.

Female mentees have also been known to manipulate their male mentors and trainers to do their bidding like accommodating their lousiness, laziness and other misdemeanours. The male mentor may succumb for fear of being labelled a chauvinist or worse still accused of sexual harassment.

Another way the female mentee may manipulate the male mentor or trainer is to hide under the cloak of pregnancy, child birth or raising children to be irresponsible and lazy. These types of Residents and House Officers become truant and negligent doctors and as such should not be condoned. As trainees/ mentees, they are always full of excuses, lousy at assignments and unable to meet deadlines. It is possible for a woman to have children and still hold her own and do the expected. Of a truth, pregnancy, child birth and raising children are challenging and time consuming responsibilities. However, it is possible to create a healthy and an effective balance bearing in mind that all others also have one challenge or another in their personal lives. Your own personal responsibility or challenge therefore should not be used to manipulate and blackmail others. More so, a lot of women have also gone through the same challenges while in Medical Profession. In fact, one of my Residents in Internal Medicine had a set of triplets and nursed them without being lazy at work. She was successful in her examinations and is at par with her contemporaries in the required posting. Granted, there were times when her colleagues and trainers accommodated her but then, she was never manipulative. She is a good example of how to behave in the face of a challenge.

There are other ways in which the mentee or trainee can constantly emotionally manipulate the mentor or trainer. This is commonly done in Nigeria in view of our diversity. The first way is when an undeserving trainee/mentee expects an unmerited approval or recommendation by the mentor since they come from the same ethnic group or are of the same religion. The mentor may give him the needed recommendation for fear of being derided by his own ethnic group.

A further way is when the undeserving trainee may manipulate the mentor or trainer by attributing the trainer's disapproval to the fact that both of them are not from the same state, ethnic group or religion. Such persons are cry babies that play ethnicity or religion as their trump card. This is sheer blackmail and should be discouraged.

Some of these manipulations should be handled during the training for the mentors. The roles of the mentors should be clearly defined. Moreover, mentors are supposed to be role models and should behave in a respectful manner. They should also be honest and straight forward such that their principles are known by all. In the same vein, the mentees are also taught to be responsible for their part in the programme irrespective of the challenges in their personal lives. This is the essence of books like this one.

Resentment or Jealousy from Others

Mentoring can be misunderstood if not properly defined. This is especially so when the mentor and mentee are of the opposite sex. The spouse of either may get jealous and resent all the time his or her spouse spends with the mentor or mentee. This can cause some degree of marital disharmony in either the mentor or mentees marriage

In addition, in organizations with developed formal Mentoring programmes, mentoring is a much sought after activity because of its positive effect on people's professional development. Be that as it may, many Mentoring programmes cannot include everyone. This causes a lot of resentments from those who did not have the opportunity to participate in the programme.

Some of the peers either criticize the program or express their resentment regularly. The resentment is also very obvious when the mentee can get ahead in many issues because of the network of his mentor. In some cases, some people believe that their peer has a better or more available mentor and as such more gains. In Nigeria, this could be in the area of job appointments, recommendation for grants and other such gains. Other peers feel that they missed out because there was not a level play ground leading to resentment.

The issue of the jealousy of the spouse is best solved by involving the spouses from the beginning of the process and defining the boundaries of the mentoring relationship in a way that they understand. Some of the meetings could be held in open places or even in homes where the spouse is in attendance and may even participate in the conversation. The practice of Mentoring circles is helpful in defining boundaries and preventing jealousy from spouses.

The jealousy of the other Residents or trainees may not be easy to deal with but such Residents may benefit from peer mentoring where their more opportune colleagues share some of their experiences with them. They should also learn to appreciate their own developments and gains from their own different mentoring programmes albeit informal? In addition Mentoring circles also handle the problem o having few mentors and many mentees.

CHAPTER 9

THE MYTHS OF MENTORING

"I believe in destiny but I also believe that you just can't sit back and let destiny happen".

Spike Lee

The concept of Mentoring has been clouded with many myths that make it undesirable or unimportant in many climes. Some of the myths are discussed below.

The Myth of Not Needed
There are some persons who believe that they do not need a mentor. They can be their own mentor and so can any other person. Considering the fact that you are reading this book, then thank God that you are not one of such. Everyone needs a mentor and everyone has been mentored by some person or persons albeit informally. We have all had parents or older relatives, friends, teachers, trainers, senior colleagues and all who made significant impacts in our lives. Formal mentoring as earlier noted is needed in order to have great achievements. Everybody needs to be mentored and also needs to mentor others at some time or another in their career or life.

The Myth of Age
In most cases, the mentor is usually an older or a senior member of the profession. This has led to the belief that the mentor is generally older than the mentee. Some others feel that they do not qualify to be a mentor since they are still relatively young. Much as the mentor is usually older and senior in the profession or the organization, this is not always so. The mentor or trainer can be older or younger. It

is not about age rather it is about having the desired knowledge, skills and experiences that will enhance the mentee. This issue of age and seniority has caused some friction especially in the cases of doctors who came for residency or further training some years later than their contemporaries. As at the time they commenced the residency training, they find that their trainers and mentors are either their peers or even younger. Some of these trainees or mentees have caused trouble by looking down on the trainer solely because of age; a good number have issues with insubordination, disobedience and arrogance. Such trainees are difficult to teach and mentor.

It is worthy of note that personally I consider Dr Udeme Ekrikpo (Consultant Nephrologist) my mentor in authorship albeit informally. Dr Ekrikpo is not only younger than me in age; he is also junior to me in the hierarchy. He is my Cheerleader and has consistently encouraged me to write. I am an author today because of his unfailing support. That is the essence of Mentoring; it is about getting the needed guidance for the mentee's professional development.

Another common scenario may occur in cases where some ethnic groups generally consider women inferior to men. This is common in some ethnic groups in Nigeria. Having a woman as the senior colleague and as such the trainer or mentor has led to insubordination and failure of mentoring and training. This is very wrong and the mentee will be the looser; of course. Mentoring is about acquiring the needed knowledge and skills to enhance the mentees career development irrespective of the age and gender of the mentor.

The Myth of Seniority
Most mentors as earlier noted are both senior and older, however, this is not exactly so. The mentor must not necessarily be senior to the mentee in the organization or

the profession. It is true that mentoring programmes always match a senior and a junior person in the mentoring pair considering that the senior has more knowledge, skills and experience than the mentee. In informal mentoring, the mentor may be junior to the mentor. The emphasis is on the needs of the mentee at such a time. Hence one can mentor his peers or his seniors as in peer or situational mentoring. In peer mentoring someone can guide his own colleague because he is passing through similar issues and is more likely to communicate at the same level.

In some other cases, the system may have changed a bit or drastically and only the peers are able to relate what the trainee is going through. One typical example in the Nigerian Residency training is the clinical examinations organized by the post graduate colleges as part of the examinations. Traditionally for many decades, the clinical examinations were in the format of long cases and short cases. In essence, this was the format of clinical examination that most of the Consultants took during their training. Currently however, the Post Graduate Colleges have adopted the more modern Objective Structured Clinical Examination (OSCE). This new format has made it difficult for the trainers and mentors to guide their Residents and techniques on examination techniques. The onus lies on the other Residents and junior Consultants who are familiar with the new format to guide both the Residents and the older Consultants. This is not only a type of peer mentoring but also the juniors mentoring the seniors (situational mentoring). Mentoring is not about seniority.

Another type of situational Mentoring occurs when an expert in a particular field comes to train and guide in the institution. Some of these could be the use of E-Library, internet services or security workshops. The mentor or trainee does not have to be senior to the trainees or mentees. This also occurs after a junior member of the department has gone for a special training (DOTS, PMTCT etc). He or she is expected to train all others irrespective of the fact that most of them are senior to him.

The Myth of Same Profession or Specialty
Mentors are usually role models that the mentee is required to follow for guidance. However, in some cases, the mentor and mentee may not necessarily be in the same profession of specialty. As a medical doctor, I can inspire, motivate or guide young people to get a university education. They don't all have to be medical doctors like myself; that will be making them my puppets. My role is to identify or recognize their own innate abilities, potentials and passions and guide them accordingly. My mentee can be an accountant, photographer or an architect based on my understanding of the person and his skills. It is always better to bloom where you are planted. We cannot all be the same. For those in the same profession with me, they do not have to be in my subspecialty. I am an Internist (Neurologist) but my mentee can be an Obstetrician, or an Ophthalmologist. Even those who are Internists do not have to be Neurologists. I need to observe where their strengths are. In some cases, the mentee may need guidance in a particular area and he or she can get the guidance from a mentor in another profession or specialty. In my university, Prof Aniekan Abasiattai (an Obstetrician) has published more than 100 papers in our setting riddled many challenges top most of which is poor or no funding at all. I always ask all those who are passionate in researches to get tips from him irrespective of their department. These mentees from other specialties do not need his surgical or obstetric skills: it is about acquiring the needed skills in prolific research.

Again, all medical doctors involved in administration and management will need guidance in the previous administrators who had occupied those positions who are not necessarily in the same department.

In addition, the mentor may not even have the ability that he sees in the mentee but will encourage such a mentee to explore that potential to the fullest. Dr Ekrikpo whom I mentioned earlier continually encouraged me to write saying that I am a good writer. He is my cheer leader despite not having the same potentials that made me an author: he was able to see those potentials in me. A mentor therefore does not have to be in the same specialty or have the same skills. Nevertheless, he or she can appreciate those qualities, skills and talents in another person.

The Myth of Being for only those in Trouble

Many people believe that only those who have problems are the ones who need mentors to guide them through the difficult times. This may be the reason that makes some people believe that they do not need a mentor because they do not have problems and can cope with their problems if any. Granted mentors as noted earlier can help the people to navigate through difficult times, mentoring is not for only those who have problems. This erroneous type of Mentoring was especially practiced when I was at the University of Port Harcourt in Nigeria. We had what was then known as Academic Advisers. Every student was assigned to a lecturer as an Academic Adviser to oversee his or her academic progress. Most of us who were supposedly good students never got to know our Academic Adviser. The Academic Advisers only sent for the bad students and those who were about to fail out. We actually thought that the role of the Academic Advisers was to advise failing students on how to change from one course to another. In retrospect, I wish that those Academic Advisers were more of what we understand today as mentors. Some of us who were supposedly good students (that were thought not to have needed them) would have benefitted immensely from guidance of some type or another.

This is to say that participating in a Mentoring programme is not a weakness, but rather a necessary tool for all professional development and as such essential for every stage of personal and professional development. The essence of a good mentor therefore is to show someone how to take the right steps to where they want to be. *Everybody who wants to develop and improve on all aspects will benefit from a mentor not just the ones in trouble.*

The Myth of Sole Benefit of Mentees
I have had senior colleagues wonder what their business with Mentoring is. This is because they believe that only mentees benefit from Mentoring. Such persons are therefore not ready to "waste their time" for something that is not beneficial to them. This conviction is not entirely correct because much as the Mentoring process is about the mentee and his progress, the mentor also has a lot of benefits. Some of these benefits for the mentor have been outlined in chapter 3 above. **Mentors have a lot to gain from the Mentoring process. In fact, as a mentor, the experience should enhance your own career development.**

One of the main advantages of mentoring young doctors is that the mentor gets challenged with new ideas. This is particularly so in the area of communications. In this new computer age, the younger generation is more versed and comfortable with the new techniques. The mentor if anything is gradually updated with the new definitions, modifications to procedures and the like. In fact one of my mentors on reviewing this book acknowledged that she had learnt a lot and also updated her skills in reviewing documents.

Mentoring also gives much respect, reverence and credibility to the mentor considering that the success of the mentee is also his or her success.

The Myth of Being Controlled

Some individuals fear that they may lose control of their personality or individuality because they wrongly believe that mentors tell you what to do and how to run your life. Granted, this fear is real because some mentors are actually Puppeteers. However, good Mentoring does not turn the mentee into a puppet. The business of the mentor is to guide and support the mentee to his or her own full potential.

Mentoring is a tool that should be used along with other types of support like didactic lectures, seminars, workshops and all. The role of the mentor is to give an outside perspective, listen and share their own experiences, give honest and constructive feedback and unbiased support and encouragement. The mentor is not supposed to tell the mentee what to do. This means that mentoring should not be controlling. It encompasses guidance, motivation, listening, challenging and providing constructive criticisms. Controlling or manipulation in any form is discouraged.

The Myth of Completion

Most formal Mentoring programmes stop when the goals of the mentee has been achieved. In informal Mentoring programmes, some also believe that Mentoring stops once the mentee becomes successful or has completed the residency training. This is not exactly true; it is akin to saying that parenting stops when the child is of a certain age. Closure may be a part of the process in the formal Mentoring programmes as already noted above. In fact, some Mentoring processes (Flash mentoring) just need only one session followed by the closure.

In some cases however, the Mentoring relationship blossoms into a beautiful friendship that lasts forever. The mentor and mentee still meet less regularly to discuss important issues or just enjoy each other's company as friends.

Again, people need different types of mentors at different times in their lives. A teenager will need a mentor to guide him into a profession or vocation in life. During his training, he needs mentors to train him in the acquisition of the necessary knowledge and skills needed for his chosen profession e.g. Academic Advisers, Lecturers and Mentors in the university. On graduation as a Medical Doctor, he needs another mentor or set of mentors to guide him through the Residency Programme. On completion, such a doctor still needs mentors to guide him in his chosen career which may be academics, management or global health and so on. He also needs mentors in his personal life, research and anything that he desires to excel in. Mentoring is an unending process: Mentoring relationships are dynamic and go through different phases over time.

The Myth of 'Godfatherism'
Mentoring has been misused in many scenarios such that the mentor represents a "godfather" or some sort of a "king maker". In this kind of relationship, the mentor or more appropriately "godfather" is a respected senior or elder who has a lot of influence where it matters and can therefore install the 'king' irrespective of whose ox is gored. This makes the supposed mentees look for those who can advance their agenda not necessarily their personal and professional development. This scenario is very common in political and executive appointments. It involves a lot of power play by the very many godfathers. The godfather takes his godson and moves him through the upper echelons of power. Thereafter, the godson remains 'loyal' to the godfather all through his tenure in the office. All or

most of his or her actions will have to be approved by the godfather; these may not necessarily be good, proper or acceptable in the setting.

The problem with this godfatherism is that the supposed Mentoring process looks more like cutting a good deal where both the mentor and mentee have their own selfish desires. It is true that Mentoring as earlier noted in most cases usually involves the introduction of the mentee to the mentor's network. This will eventually enhance the mentee such that a fast rise in the hierarchy or prestigious appointment may be part of the benefits. However, the essence of Mentoring is for personal and professional development. It is to support the mentee to release his potentials and grow to be the best that he can be not to automatically give him an exalted position.

CHAPTER 10

STARTING OFF A MENTORING PROGRAMME

"A single step is the beginning of a thousand miles".
Chinese Proverb

"The man who moves a mountain begins by carrying away small stones"
Confucius

Starting a mentoring programme like most things in life is not always easy. Starting off on a wrong footing will definitely result in the failure of the programme. The first step for a successful programme will be to convince all the key players of the need of such a programme. This will particularly require the support of the top management of the organization. The watchword still remains *preparation.* There are several challenges within this period some of which have been described above. There are many ways to start off the mentoring programme. However, I particularly like the key principles of the Training Connection's Inc which has a comprehensive and systematic approach for the take off. It has been implemented in scores of private and public organizations with immense success.

These key principles for an effective successful programme embedded in the TTC Inc are seen in Fig 8. as follows:

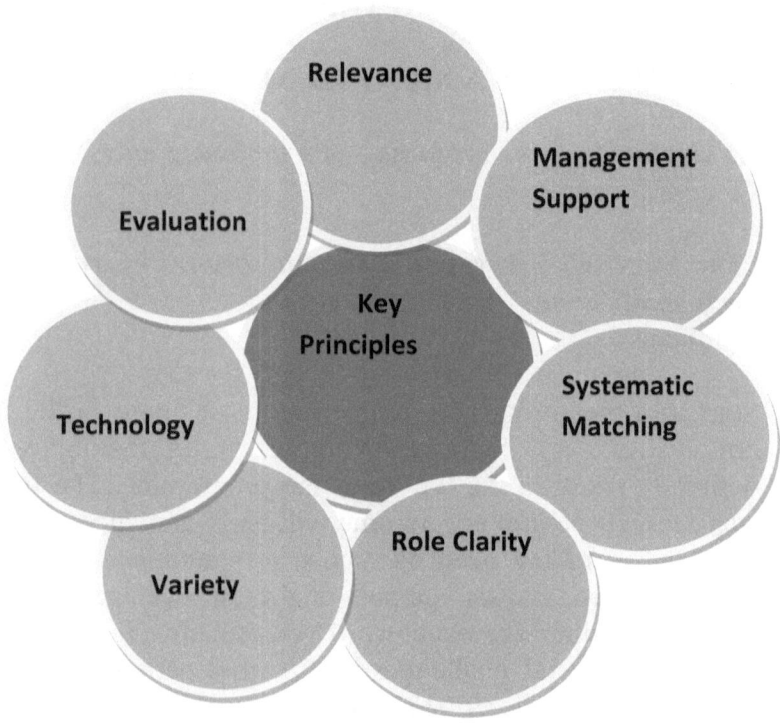

Fig 8. Key principles

Relevance

The first step in starting a Mentoring Programme is to define whether it is relevant for the institution. Having read this book to this chapter, I can assume that you consider mentoring relevant in your practice and training. Your mentoring program however will have to be designed to meet the unique needs of the practice and training in your institution. Medicine is not the same as any other profession. The training process is basically the same in most of our training programmes in the world with mild variations and modifications. As noted earlier, the

Residency Programme has two prongs; comprising a full time Medical Practice and a full time Postgraduate Training. The programme will have to be structured in a way that does not obstruct the flow of the training as well as patient care.

Top Management Support
It is pertinent for the management of the hospital to be carried along for the programme to succeed. For starters, the management may have to create the unit and appoint a programme manager. The needful trainings and tools will have to be organized and procured with the support of the management: financially and otherwise. Other line managers in the administrative hierarchy will also be involved. This will include the head of department, head of the residency training programme and the chief Resident in each department for the smooth running of the programme.

Systematic Matching
Having ensured the support of the top management staff, the next step is the recruitment of would be mentors and mentees into the programme. Thereafter these individuals are systematically and carefully matched based on their goals, visions, specialties, gender and personalities. This is the reason the line managers are involved ab initio to ensure that there are few mistakes. Most programmes permit the mentees to make an input in the choice of their mentor. In a new programme where there are few mentors, the mentoring circle is ideal.

Role Clarity
It is important that the roles and responsibilities of both the mentors and mentees are clearly defined. In that way, both of them will be better focused on the task ahead. For us in the Medical Profession, this is usually acquisition of the knowledge and skills which ultimately translate to success

in the post graduate examinations. Other areas of interest include mentoring in research, administration and leadership. The programme organizer clearly defines the roles of both the mentors and the mentees.

Variety
Another key principle that should be put in place at this time is the issue of variety. Some people in the system may not understand why they also may need to be mentored. For example, a Consultant may think that he has already being appointed having being successful in all his examinations. In essence he has no need for a mentor. He may however need a mentor in leadership, training, research, authorship and or administration. Ensuring the principle of mentoring in different areas for career development is a key principle. The Residents and trainees can also be exposed to different mentors. Variety is the spice of life and will therefore make the mentoring experience more enriching and rewarding.

Technology
Mentoring involves much communication especially face-to face communication. However, the use of telecommunication has made communication much easier in recent times. The use of telecommunication in mentoring is therefore regarded as one of the key principles. Having established the initial communication and rapport, it is recommended that the mentors and mentees may use the internet to manage some of the information. This will include regular E mails, WhatsApp and text messages.

Evaluation
Evaluation is another key principle in a formal mentoring programme. The programme design therefore must include a time for evaluation. This evaluation should be carried out periodically to ascertain the progress of the programme. It is also pertinent to assess whether the goals of the

programme are being achieved. Good progress and the achievement of the goals connote a successful programme. Whereas, the lack of progress or non achievement of the goals may lead to the final phase of mentoring: the conclusion. Conclusion may also come when all the goals have been achieved and it is time for the mentee to move on or change to another type of mentor. The programme therefore should be designed to ensure the principles listed above are included in the mentoring programme.

Suggested Steps for the hospital

Plan the Program's Purpose and Design
The hospitals should set up a small committee or unit which will include the residency training coordinator of the hospital. This committee should be headed by the Chairman, Medical Advisory committee who is also the Head of Clinical Services. It may be better to start off in the different departments in the institutions which are new at the programme to test the waters. Eventually the different systems from the different programmes will merge into a bigger programme for the hospital having overcome some of the teething problems.

Identify the Potential Mentors and Mentees
Everybody may not be interested in mentoring. Some others however who are interested may not be available for the programme. It is therefore pertinent to identify individuals who are interested and are also available for the mentoring programme. This will make the programme start off strong with committed and available mentors.

Facilitate an Orientation Programme
There should be an orientation programme or workshop for all the stake holders. This will include the mentors, mentees and the supervisors. The importance of training and retraining cannot be overemphasized.

Match the Mentors and Mentees
This is an extremely important step in the Mentoring process. This will take into consideration their specialties, personalities and individual strengths. Other considerations include their different methods of studying, their clinical itinerary. It is also better if the mentees chose their mentors based on the qualities they see in them. Again mentoring circle is recommended where there are few mentors

Implementation
The mentoring process is then commenced. This is usually not easy like most good things in life. There will be challenges at every step that need to be circumvented. It will need work, work and more work.

Evaluation and Tracking
The programme requires tracking and regular evaluations. Some mentoring pairs may have to be changed and reassigned. Some individuals may drop out of the programme based on their increased work load and availability. There may need to redesign some aspects of the programme. The programme will take time to meet your Mentoring needs.

Finding a Mentor

Anyone who is interested in career development needs a mentor as already noted. Formal mentoring is highly recommended in all hospitals and training institutions. However, in situations where there is no formal mentoring programme, individuals who want to be mentored can still go ahead on their own. Such persons will need to choose their mentors whom they believe will enhance them. Below are some of the important tips in finding suitable mentors.

Reach Out

Sometimes *far* out Mentorship can be found in an infinite number of places at healthcare training institutions. This depends on what the mentee needs to achieve. The mentor may even be in a different hospital, different setting or specialty. For example a Resident who desires to have a career administration and management can reach out to a medical doctor who is an administrator in the Health Services in Health Management Board. Some of my mentors like my Cheerleader Dr Mfon Edyang–Ekpa are not in the same specialty of health system with me. Dr Charles Amanari who has been the Librarian that furnished me with so much information and resources is a Plastic Surgeon while I am an internist. Please do not be afraid to reach out across other specialties and institutions.

Use the Full Spectrum

Mentors exist at all stages of the medical career—not just at the top. Thus, you should work to find peer mentors at all stages, including those just beginning their careers and those who are very well accomplished in your area of interest. As a medical student or House Officer (intern) you need peer mentors and also junior Residents to acquire basic knowledge and clinical skills. This will help you to achieve goals like success in your examinations, successful houseman ship and practice during the National Youth Service Corps (NYSC). As a Resident, you also need peer mentors, then senor Registrars and Consultants to acquire more knowledge and improve your clinical skills; This will lead to success in the postgraduate examinations, increased confidence in clinical and surgical skills and in due course being appointed a Consultant. As a Consultant, you need peer mentoring and mentoring by the senior Consultant in the area of research, leadership, administration and so on. *In essence, at every point in time during your training, you will achieve more with a mentor.*

Sub specialize your mentors
All medical doctors have lots of balls to juggle. These include clinical pursuits, research projects, career and personal development activities. All these are superimposed your personal life, responsibilities and challenges. It is therefore wise to select different mentors for different aspects of your career development. The more, the merrier and you will be richer for it.

Quality control
Quality is more important than quantity. First and foremost, a mentor should be someone who makes time for the mentee. Such a person should inspire you to be a better doctor and a better person through their example and advice. It is difficult for an absentee irrespective of his or her level of knowledge and experience to make an impact. Be sure to choose someone that has time for you.

Return the favour
It is never too early to become a mentor. You can be a good peer-mentor to your fellow Residents and medical students (also known as a good friend), a teacher and confidant for your junior Residents and an inspiration to your medical students. The sooner you start the better for you.

CONCLUSION

Informal Mentoring has been practiced in all organizations, institutions and a wide variety of businesses. Formal Mentoring however is novel and has been called the sine qua non of Management considering the immense benefits. The dire need for the implementation of Formal Mentoring programmes in all organizations therefore cannot be overemphasized. This is more so in the hectic Medical Practice and Training. Starting off a mentoring programme is never easy as some of the challenges have been outlined. However, the gains are numerous and as such make tackling the enormous challenges worthwhile.
Formal Mentoring should therefore also be the sine qua non of the Medical Profession.

"We rise by lifting others".
Robert Ingersoll

REFERENCES

1. https://en.wikipedia.org/wiki/Mentoring

2. https://www.management-mentors.com/resources/benefits-of-Mentoring

3. https://www.irishtimes.com/life-and-style/people/ann-ward-pioneering-Obstetrician-and-missionary-nun-1.2698516

4. https://ed4online.com/blog/9-types-mentors-have-your-lifes

5. https://www.kaptest.com/blog/residency-secrets/2016/06/29/finding-mentors-in-your-medical-career-file:///C:/Users/USER/Documents/The%20Mentoring%20Process.html

6. http://www.halorecognition.com/the-huge-importance-of-mentors-in-developing-top-talent/https://www.management-mentors.com/about/corporate-mentoring-matters-blog/bid/64145/Mentoring-Circle

7. Malu A O. Universities and Medical Education in Nigeria. Niger Med J 2010:51:2, 84-88

8. Ramani S, Grippe L, Kocher Eke. Twelve tips for developing effective mentors. Medical Teacher, Vol. 28, No. 5, 2006, pp. 404–408

Dr Bertha Chioma Ekeh is a Senior Lecturer and Consultant Neurologist in University of Uyo/University of Uyo Teaching Hospital (UUTH) in Nigeria. She has a passion for Teaching, Training and Mentoring and is currently the Coordinator of Residency Training in the Hospital.

Other books by Dr Bertha Chioma Ekeh

Clinical Neurology Made Easy
Fundamentals of Neurological Diagnosis
Textbook of Neurology
Principles of Prosperity

www.ingramcontent.com/pod-product-compliance
Lightning Source LLC
Chambersburg PA
CBHW031435210526
45464CB00005B/2218